Lois Halzel Freedman, MEd

Birth As a Healing Experience
The Emotional Journey of Pregnancy Through Postpartum

Pre-publication
REVIEW

"**M**s. Freedman's book gives insight into the emotions involved with pregnancy and loss. Her sensitivity and unique ability to break through emotional roadblocks pertaining to birth, and guide women to a place of healing, is a gift.

The stories of the women are fascinating—their relevance to what is the 'medical cultural norm' gives childbirth educators and health care providers an awareness of the power of their words and actions, as it pertains to this most important life transition."

Mary E. Baker, BSN, CNM, CCE
Certified Nurse Midwife,
Wellesley Women's Care,
Wellesley, MA

Birth As a Healing Experience
The Emotional Journey of Pregnancy Through Postpartum

HAWORTH Innovations in Feminist Studies
J. Dianne Garner
Senior Editor

Birth As a Healing Experience
The Emotional Journey of Pregnancy Through Postpartum

Lois Halzel Freedman, MEd

The Haworth Press
New York • London • Oxford

The Haworth Press, Inc., 10 Alice Street, Binghamton, NY 13904-1580

Cover design by Dianne Hodack.

Library of Congress Cataloging-in-Publication Data

Freedman, Lois Halzel.
    Birth as a healing experience : the emotional journey of pregnancy through postpartum / Lois Halzel Freedman.
        p.   cm.
    Includes bibliographical references and index.
    ISBN 0-7890-0576-X (alk. paper)
    1. Pregnancy—Psychological aspects. 2. Puerperium—Psychological aspects. I. Title.
RG560.F74 1999
618.2′001′9—dc21   99-16075
                                                                                            CIP

To my children, Scott and Melissa,
whose births changed my life
and led me to pursue my career,
which is as close to my heart
as are both of you.

ABOUT THE AUTHOR

Lois Halzel Freedman, MEd, is a certified childbirth educator with fifteen years of experience in the field of prenatal and postpartum support. Currently, she has a private practice in individual prenatal and postpartum counseling. Ms. Freedman also facilitates individual and group childbirth education classes, vaginal birth after cesarean (VBAC) preparation series, postpartum women's series, and provides individual labor support. She specializes in helping women heal from past loss and trauma as they prepare for childbirth and enter the postpartum period. Ms. Freedman is a consultant in the field of prenatal and postpartum education, having lectured at community health centers and other community-based programs. In 1997, she gave a presentation entitled "Compassionate Childbirth Preparation" to physicians at a women's maternity hospital in Moscow, Russia. Ms. Freedman lives in the Boston area with her husband and two teenage children.

CONTENTS

Foreword

I come to the writing of the foreword for Lois Halzel Freedman's book from many perspectives. As coordinator of a pregnancy/environmental hotline, I counseled women for eleven years about the potential risks to pregnancy and the fetus from commonly occurring exposures such as medications and chemicals. In addition, I am a motherless mother and a friend and relative to many women who have had their babies by cesarean section. Perhaps most important, as Lois's friend and colleague, I have witnessed and assisted at the birth of this book.

In my work at the hotline, I was often struck by the level of anxiety experienced by so many pregnant women who called the service. Why were they so worried about sometimes the most trivial of exposures— to plant food, chemical additives, or Tylenol? I recognized then that it was not always the substances that concerned them but rather their general fears about the pregnancy, the baby, and labor. For many women, placing their fears in the rational, scientific context of something they thought they could control, namely exposures, provided relief from their ambient anxiety. Since all pregnant women come into contact with something of potential concern, services such as the hotline are extremely valuable. It was clear to me, however, that these women needed to talk and be listened to, to have their fears taken seriously, and that this did not always occur in the offices of their care providers.

This book will help those who provide health care and education to pregnant women to recognize and honor the importance of their clients' emotional lives. One of the important lessons in Lois's book is that all women need empathic support during pregnancy and the postpartum time. For women who had traumatic birth experiences such as an unexpected cesarean section, this support is even more critical. Lois does not suggest that all care providers of pregnant and postpartum women take on the role of a friendly therapist. However, the hope is that more physicians, nurses, midwives, therapists, and childbirth educators will adopt an openness and awareness of the tenderness of this time for many women, that they will listen to women, and where appropriate, refer them to a compassionate and knowledgeable childbirth professional.

I lost my mother to cancer when I was nineteen and she forty-five. To say that the loss of my mother at such an early age was very painful is an understatement. Like many of Lois's clients, I sought help to deal with that loss. Though I had the support of a caring family, when I became pregnant and a new mother, the well of emptiness of not having my own mother there to love and dote on me and my babies felt like a great chasm. A new level of grief was exposed.

For my first pregnancy, my husband and I chose the care of a hospital-based nurse-midwifery practice. Toward the end of the pregnancy, for administrative reasons, the practice moved to the hospital in which my mother had died twelve years earlier. The location of this hospital was far from my home and we decided to change to another midwifery practice in a hospital more conveniently located.

I also knew that I could not deliver at that hospital. The memories of my mother's last days there were still vivid. I remember feeling that the birth of my baby could not possibly occur where I had lost my mother. I felt that something terrible might happen. Though this seemed somewhat foolish, irrational, and superstitious at the time, I knew that I needed to follow my instincts. As much as I cherished my first midwife, and experienced leaving her as a loss, I knew I had made the correct choice for that pregnancy. It might have eased that time for me had I been able to read the writing and stories in Lois's book, to know that I was not alone in these fears and feelings.

For me, the postpartum and new motherhood time presented the greatest challenges. I found that time difficult, longing for the support and advice of my mother in ways I had never imagined. It was not until reading Lois's book that I fully appreciated the effect of early mother loss on my ability to become a mother myself. Reading about Lois's work with women, I know that the support they received helped in their transformation from motherless daughters to motherless mothers. Their stories validated my own struggles and helped in my own growth and healing.

I was fortunate to have two natural births and two healthy children. I see now that, without knowing it, I followed the suggestions

Lois makes in Chapter 5. I had wonderful support from my husband and midwives. Most important, I felt empowered by my choices and respected by my caregivers. The guidelines in this book are invaluable to anyone planning for a fulfilling birth experience.

Lois Freedman shares her vision of birth as a time when a woman and her partner deserve to feel well-informed, nurtured, and empowered. She outlines the state of cesarean section in this country, describing the "medicalization of childbirth." Lois balances the need for and uses of technology with the possibilities of female-centered childbirth. For pregnant women and their partners, information is given to assist in making appropriate choices for their births.

It is Lois's intention that anyone who reads her book will have a heightened sensitivity to the breadth of emotions brought on during pregnancy, birth, and postpartum. The stories of her clients are the heart of the book and speak to the heart of the reader. They showcase the possibilities for transformation during this precious time in a woman's life.

Susan Kepnes Rosenwasser, MEd
Sharon, MA

Preface

My interest in the field of childbirth preparation began with the birth of my son, Scott, by cesarean section seventeen years ago. I went on to have a vaginal birth after cesarean with my second child, Melissa, two years later. Within a few months of my second child's birth, I began my studies through the Boston Association for Childbirth Education, attending classes and births, reading numerous childbirth books, and preparing to become a Certified Childbirth Educator. My inspiration from my two remarkably different birth experiences gave me insight and an ability to relate to pregnant women and their partners. After teaching childbirth classes as a Certified Childbirth Educator for several years, I furthered my studies at Lesley College, where I received a master's degree in education with a specialty in childbirth education.

As a childbirth educator and counselor, I am honored to be part of the circle of women providing love and assistance to a woman and her partner during this major life transition. I have helped women and couples prepare for birth, give birth, and have supported them in the adjustment after their babies were born. In my work, I acknowledge that giving birth is a sacred life experience to be honored by all those who are involved with or working with women. The period from pregnancy through postpartum is an important developmental stage in a woman's life. This time presents a special opportunity for women to explore the many emotional issues that may arise as a result of the profound act of bearing and giving birth to a new being.

While my focus is on the experience of women during pregnancy through the postpartum period, I would like to acknowledge that the woman's partner plays a very important and active part in the preparation for birth and in the actual birth experience. Those who participate in supportive roles lend tremendous strength to the pregnant and laboring woman. Detailed information about the woman's partner is not included in this book because my work has centered on birth preparation from the childbearing woman's perspective. Although I address my writing to the pregnant and postpartum woman, much of the information in this book is applicable to her partner as well.

During childbirth preparation with my clients, I have found that a woman's unresolved experiences of loss may affect not only her birthing experience and her life as a new mother, but also her development as an adult woman. Moreover, I have discovered that women can also heal emotional wounds with the support of an empathic caregiver such as a childbirth educator or counselor.

This book explores the scholarly research about childbirth and presents my own personal experiences and stories of my clients. My hope is that its readers will be enlightened to new ways of approaching this period in a woman's life and, for those who have suffered earlier unresolved losses, to the possibility of emotional healing during pregnancy, birth, and postpartum. In this book, I tell some of the women's stories that I have been privileged to hear and also share general information and numerous conversations I have had over the years with women in my practice. All names and sufficient details have been changed to protect their confidentiality. The stories illustrate various challenges women face during pregnancy and the postpartum period, and the importance of receiving support during these times. These moving, triumphant tales have a great deal to teach us.

When I began writing this book, I intended it for women and men in their childbearing years and for professionals who assist women during pregnancy, birth, and the postpartum period. These professionals include, but are not limited to, childbirth educators, labor assistants, doulas, midwives, nurses, nurse practitioners, obstetricians, pediatricians, family practice physicians, and mental health professionals. The book that has evolved, however, has taken a broader perspective that could be interesting to any woman who is or plans to become pregnant, her partner, and anyone who has a desire to learn about the potential for personal growth and healing through the experience of childbirth. It is also of interest to a woman seeking to deal with issues related to childbearing even years after the event.

SPECIAL NOTE

This book offers information and support to women and their partners. It is not a substitute for the personalized care of a qualified health care provider. Women should discuss individual concerns with these professionals. With the exception of the author's story, all names and sufficient details have been changed to protect the identities of individuals whose stories are found in this book.

Acknowledgments

I am grateful to all of the pregnant and postpartum women whom I have helped with the physical, emotional, and spiritual aspects of giving birth. Educating you during prenatal sessions, providing assistance during childbirth, and listening to your birth stories have all enriched my experience of writing this book. It is my good fortune to have worked with many wonderful women and men. I admire and appreciate your courage to share not only the joy but also the pain of your birth experiences with me. Your stories have touched my heart and I thank you for allowing me to be a part of your lives.

I have had the privilege of being supported in this book-writing process by many friends and relatives too numerous to mention. As I have gone through the process of birthing this book, I have often envisioned myself surrounded by a large circle of people who know and love me. This is exactly what I tell pregnant women as they prepare for the birth of their baby. Encircle yourself with those who can be loving and gentle with you as you approach this very significant experience of your life—giving birth.

In pursuing my dream of writing this book, I have relied on the support of my labor assistants from whom I have drawn so much strength: Susan Rosenwasser, for her loving support, friendship, inspiration, constant encouragement, and outstanding editing. Pat Daniel, for her detailed feedback on the manuscript, and kind words of wisdom. Linky Strassman, for her body work, not only on my feet, but on my spirit. Miriam Greenspan, for all of her tender loving care, and for being the "grandmother of the book." Nancy Wainer Cohen, for being the pioneer of the VBAC movement, and for her friendship and encouragement through the years.

I am grateful to two special friends for their behind-the-scenes coaching: Rosy Granoff for encouraging me to attend graduate school, and for suggesting I keep detailed records all those long years ago; and Cindy Marcus for unique insights and for always being just a phone call away.

Many thanks also to my thesis team, Peggy Wright, Marliese Vogel, and Gail Ballester for their work on the earlier version of this book; Pat Harvey for editing expertise; and Cliff Hochman for legal assistance. I would like to acknowledge The Haworth Press and its supportive staff for launching this book into the world.

My great appreciation goes to the lay and nurse midwives with whom I have had the opportunity to work for their dedicated, gentle, and respectful care of birthing women. I am grateful to the nurses, childbirth educators, and labor support providers for their generous and kind care of pregnant women. I would also like to acknowledge all other care providers of pregnant women who honor the childbirth experience.

I thank my parents, Barbara and Isadore Halzel, for the love and genuine interest and pride they have shown in my work over the years. Thanks to my sisters, Cindy Levy and Amy Willis, for their enthusiasm and many hours on the phone, to my in-laws, Ann and Maynard Freedman, for their love and words of support.

Thanks to my children, Scott and Melissa, now both teenagers, for believing in me, being my biggest fans, encouraging me when I needed it, and helping me with the computer during the writing of this book. They have taught me about humor, love, and the joy of being their mother.

I thank my husband, Arnold, for all the support, love, and patience he has so generously offered as I labored to finish this project. When I wanted to have a baby without medical intervention, he was my greatest proponent. Years later, when I was sure I could not proceed any further with this book, he reminded me that I could do anything I set out to do. His sense of humor and delicious meals have gotten me through many a dark moment. Special thanks for believing in my abilities and enthusiastically encouraging me to pursue my dreams.

PART I:
BIRTH AS PERSONAL
AND PSYCHOLOGICAL DEVELOPMENT

Chapter 1

The Author's Own Story:
Two Births and One Book

Perhaps wisdom is simply a matter of waiting, and healing a question of time.

Rachel Naomi Remen
Kitchen Table Wisdom
1996, p. 333

BIRTH NUMBER ONE

On March 13, 1982, I gave birth by cesarean section to a beautiful, healthy, six-pound, twelve-ounce boy in a large Boston teaching hospital. Little did I know the impact this event would have on my life. I was an educated, informed, physically fit young woman. I received thorough prenatal care from an obstetrician who was affiliated with this hospital. My husband and I attended the childbirth education classes at the hospital, as was suggested by my physician. When the childbirth educator showed a film about cesarean section, I was sure I would not need a cesarean because I was healthy and my pregnancy was normal. During prenatal visits, I asked my doctor questions about labor and he assured me that everything would be fine. I was told not to worry. I assumed I would be assisted by him.

I went into labor on March 10. After I labored at home for two days, my husband and I decided to go to the hospital because I was having painful contractions that were coming steadily every five to seven minutes. The physician admitted me and performed an internal examination. He suggested that we go home because I was only dilated two centimeters. What would I do at home when it was hurting so much already? My husband and I thought that in the hospital I would have the support of the hospital staff. We decided to stay.

During my long labor in the hospital, I was quite surprised that I saw my physician infrequently. Shifts of nurses came and went. During the long hours of labor I was not allowed to eat or drink. I was given ice chips for nourishment and Pitocin to speed up my "slow labor." I underwent many internal exams, and was given an epidural to eliminate the pain. Eventually I had to be given IV fluids to avoid becoming dehydrated after this length of time laboring in the hospital. I felt scared, wondering why my labor was proceeding so slowly. I felt alone. Although my husband stayed with me and helped me breathe through every contraction, he did not know why they kept telling us that it was taking a very long time for me to have this baby. Neither of us had any idea of the powerlessness that we would both feel while I labored for so many hours in the impersonal hospital room. Finally, after about twenty-four hours, I was told that I was now ready to start to push my baby out. After pushing for two hours I felt exhausted and defeated. My obstetrician told me it was time to perform a cesarean section. The baby was doing fine, but he decided my labor had gone on long enough. I was very disappointed to not have a "normal birth" and slightly relieved to be finished with this painful, frightening ordeal.

My baby was delivered by cesarean section. Right after he was taken from my abdomen, I was told that he was a healthy baby boy. At that time, I asked my husband a number of times if the baby was healthy. Although I know he told me repeatedly that our baby looked fine, I felt uncertain because I did not see him or hold him. I did not see my son until many hours after the birth. In the recovery room, I remember my mother coming in to see me as I awoke from the surgery. She told me that the baby was fine, and reassured me that I would be fine too. I did not feel fine. I remember feeling detached from my son and from the information about him. After the birth I felt sick and very weak. I did not have any idea then that I could have taken more responsibility for this most powerful event of my life.

When I asked my physician why I had needed a cesarean section, he replied that my labor was too long and I was not able to push my baby out. The medical terms for this are numerous: dystocia, failure to progress, or cephalopelvic disproportion (CPD). I know today that my labor was quite long, but that this fact alone is not a reason for a cesarean. I had pushed for two hours after I had been given epidural anesthesia. Because of the consequent loss of sensation and muscle control, I was not free to change my position to help the baby be born. I was told that, because I had pushed long and unsuccessfully, it had been necessary for me to have a cesarean. I felt like a failure.

Months later, I was still tired, physically uncomfortable, and emotionally exhausted. Here I was with this beautiful healthy baby boy, yet I was not able to fully enjoy my role as a new mother. I could not have imagined that my birthing experience would have such an impact on my ability to mother him and to appreciate the gifts in my life. It took me a full year to recover physically and emotionally from the unexpected abdominal surgery that I had endured to give birth.

THE SECOND BABY:
PRACTICING THE LESSONS LEARNED

When my son was in his second year of life, I became pregnant again. Because of the difficulty of the first birth, I began to explore the process of childbirth and its alternatives. I knew I did not want another cesarean section unless it was absolutely necessary. I did not want to undergo surgery to have my next baby. When I inquired, my obstetrician stated that he thought I could probably have a vaginal birth after a cesarean. He added, however, that if I were his wife he would tell me to have another cesarean. This comment enraged me and I knew then that I needed to change obstetricians.

After consulting with Nancy Wainer Cohen, the author of *Silent Knife* (Cohen and Estner, 1983) and pioneer of the vaginal birth after cesarean (VBAC) movement, I changed physicians during my fourth month of pregnancy. Finding an obstetrician who was willing to begin from the premise that my body was strong, healthy, and capable of giving birth naturally felt like a victory. I had learned from Nancy that it is generally preferable to change facilities from the one where the cesarean occurred when trying to have a VBAC because a woman tends to feel safer laboring and giving birth in a new location. This doctor attended all of his VBAC births at the same hospital where I had undergone my cesarean. Although it meant returning to the same hospital, we chose to continue with the new physician.

My husband and I decided to take Nancy's psychologically based VBAC course. I proceeded with my soul-searching, my thinking about the upcoming birth. I knew that I did not want another cesarean section unless it was absolutely necessary. I was determined to understand my choices and responsibilities so that I could do everything possible to avoid an unnecessary cesarean. I wanted a healthy baby as well as a fulfilling birth experience. In the course, we received a great deal of information to help us avoid an unnecessary cesarean. We talked in the group about our feelings regarding our experiences of having under-gone a cesarean. Some of us cried, and some expressed anger and a range of other feelings about our past birthing experiences. Many believed their cesareans were not necessary, but felt that at the time they had no choice. Nancy told us that none of us was a failure for having our babies by cesarean section.

Nancy emphasized that pregnant women's bodies are strong and healthy. If given enough time and support in labor, she assured us that the great majority of women are able to have vaginal births. She also stressed that giving birth vaginally after a cesarean is safer than having a repeat cesarean. She pointed out that most babies are also strong during the birthing process. At her suggestion I read informative child-birth books that further developed my confidence in my ability to give birth naturally. She encouraged us to seek out the support of a labor assistant, a woman who is trained to assist women and their partners during labor.

My husband and I hired Marilyn, a certified childbirth educator and labor assistant. We arranged for her to come to our home while I was in early labor, to help me stay at home as long as possible. She did not take the place of my husband, but rather provided support for both of us. Marilyn inspired me, reminding me I was strong and would be able to give birth vaginally. She encouraged me to allow the labor to take as long as necessary and not to be frightened or discouraged by the length and intensity of my labor. She assured me that it was not unusual for VBAC women to labor for many hours.

My labor began on July 3, 1984. Very early that morning I woke up having contractions and called Marilyn, who offered to come to my home. My son was picked up by his grandparents, who were over-joyed to spend time with him while I was in labor.

After Marilyn ascertained that I was indeed in labor, she left, giving me and my husband the opportunity to spend the day at home. We walked miles that day by a beautiful lake near our home, stopping every time I had a contraction. During each contraction I leaned on my husband in a bear hug stance. We had a pleasant, relaxing day together; I felt strong and excited that my baby was going to come soon. Months after I gave birth, people commented that they were surprised to see me that day walking miles from my home, especially since my due date had been the previous week.

By 9:00 p.m. my labor had become more intense. We called Marilyn, who came back to our house at midnight and stayed overnight. With this labor, I did not want to arrive at the hospital too early. Marilyn listened often to my baby with her fetoscope and assured me the baby's heartbeat was strong, and the baby was doing just fine. She and my husband took turns massaging my back all through the night as I continued to have contractions every five minutes.

In the morning, although I did not feel particularly hungry, Marilyn encouraged me to eat breakfast. After eating I had an urge to push, so we decided it was time to go to the hospital. Marilyn examined me at that time. I was dilated five centimeters and having contractions every three to five minutes. It was now July 4, Independence Day. We encountered a traffic jam in the center of our small town and had a police escort through town. We were finally off to Boston.

Upon entering the hospital, my labor slowed down considerably. I no longer had an urge to push. I was admitted and placed under the care of a staff obstetrician who referred to me during our initial en-counter as a "previous cesarean." I was not happy to be given this title, an impersonal reference with serious medical implications. There was nothing medically wrong with me; I had simply had an operation to have my first baby. Now I was a healthy pregnant woman. I was afraid this label meant they were going to treat me like a sick patient.

After an examination by this physician, my labor stopped com-pletely. It seemed that the entrance to this facility where I had pre-viously had my cesarean, being greeted as a medical high-risk patient, and the medicinal odors of the hospital increased my fear and halted my labor. I wanted to leave and asked my husband to contact my own obstetrician.

My obstetrician arrived shortly after being called in and, though he did not give me formal "permission" to leave the hospital, we left after signing out AMA (against medical advice). He could not give me permission to leave, even though my labor had stopped, because I was a VBAC and, therefore, considered by standard medical protocol to be at risk for a possible problem in labor. My only problem at the time was not having contractions during the active stage of labor. My baby was doing fine.

We informed my obstetrician that we were leaving for Marilyn's home, which was close to the hospital, in order for my labor to begin again. We agreed to return once I was having regular contractions.

Marilyn assured me that I would go back into labor, which I did as soon as we walked out of the hospital and into the parking lot. My contractions began to come frequently and increased during the ride to Marilyn's home. Once there, she gave my husband and me a light meal. She left us alone to labor in her living room. A few hours later, my contractions were steadily coming every three to five minutes. I was now again in active labor and felt ready to return to the hospital.

Before proceeding to the hospital, Marilyn suggested I take a shower. The shower helped relax me and gave me a little more time to labor outside of the hospital. On the ride back to the hospital, Marilyn repeatedly reassured me that I would continue to have contractions once in the hospital again, and that I could have a vaginal birth. She reminded me often during labor that my body was strong, that I could have my VBAC baby.

We arrived back at the hospital at 6:00 p.m., July 4. My cervix was dilated to seven centimeters and did not become fully dilated for another seven and a half hours. I pushed for over an hour and gave birth, free of medical interventions and medications, to a healthy girl at 2:44 a.m. July 5, 1984, in the same Boston hospital where I had experienced the cesarean two years before.

It was one of the high points of my life. I was thrilled. I felt strong and healthy after giving birth. My daughter was immediately in my arms. I looked at her, spoke to her, and was overcome with joy at having given birth to her without surgery. I felt alert and hungry, completely healthy, and pain-free. It was an exhilarating feeling. I knew I could do anything I set my mind to, now that I had given birth vaginally. The support and encouragement I received from my husband and Marilyn for those long hours meant so much to me. I had a sense of being mothered and nurtured.

BIRTH OF A CAREER AND A BOOK

Several years after having my children, I sought support from a therapist who had been recommended to me. In an early session, when she asked me about myself, I told her that the births of my children had greatly affected my life. I told her about the physical, emotional, and spiritual differences I had experienced between the first birth and the subsequent vaginal birth. I noted that I had chosen my career as a childbirth educator as a result of the pain and loss I had felt after giving birth to my first child by cesarean section.

She responded to me with surprise and confusion. I felt judged, having to explain that the cesarean birth experience brought up feelings of significant loss for me, even six years after the event. Though I shared these feelings with her, I know now that she did not understand the profound impact a cesarean section or other traumatic birth can have on a woman's life.

Later, I joined a women's support group that was facilitated by author and therapist Miriam Greenspan. Miriam immediately recognized and validated the power of the earlier birth experience and my need to heal from it. The techniques that she used in the group taught me the importance of compassion and connection in the therapeutic model. Among other objectives in writing this book, I hope to make readers aware that a traumatic experience of childbirth needs to be processed in the same way as any other major trauma. The simple telling of the birth story to a compassionate listener can begin the healing work.

I have learned from many women who shared the stories of their birthing experiences with me, some soon after giving birth and some many years later. I am always struck by how magical and profound the simple act of telling the birth story can be. For some women, it signifies strength and empowerment while for others telling the story brings up feelings of victimization, betrayal, or loss. I believe that talking about the experience of childbirth can be a valuable process for women in any stage of their lives. The stories are a legacy for future generations, and can often be the catalyst for the healing of earlier emotional and psychological damage.

While finishing the writing of this book, I had a great deal of fear of letting "my baby," this book, come out into the world. As much as I tried to let go and trust, I had tremendous anxiety. Just as I suggest that body work can be helpful to the pregnant or postpartum woman, a close friend reminded me that I might get some relief during the arduous process of finishing my book by having a body work session. I went for an appointment for reflexology* and reiki,** and had no expectations of the session except for it to be a relaxing hour. The body work practitioner, Sole Woman, had become my friend during the course of my writing.

The morning of the appointment, I had woken up with intermittent abdominal pain, which I continued to experience upon entering the session. While beginning, Sole Woman asked me how the book was coming. I told her that it was fine but that presently I was experiencing a great deal of fear. As she began to work on me, I relaxed and talked about my anxiety about my writing becoming public. I told her about my client, Sara,† whose midwives had given her plenty of time and loving encouragement during labor. I felt their patience and care had enabled Sara to give birth to her baby naturally after a long labor. At the end of our session, Sole Woman had her hand on my abdomen and she said, "Trust. It will be fine. You can push and let go." I had a memory, an image of being in the pushing stage of labor with my son. My abdomen continued to feel achy. I was hearing a gentle voice saying, "Push, you can let it go. Everything is going to be fine." My tears began to come. I lay on the table and cried.

A few moments later, I had the awareness on a very deep spiritual level that I had not had enough time to push my son, Scott, out into the world. Although I had known this for many years, I had never experienced it in quite this way before. I felt some relief and affirmation that

---

*Reflexology is the science of applying pressure to reflex points in the feet to produce a physiological effect in the body. The theory is that the foot is a mirror image of the body, a map of the stress held within the body.

**Reiki, an ancient form of Japanese healing, utilizes gentle focused touch to relax the body and encourage healing on physical, emotional, and spiritual levels.

†Sara's story appears in Chapter 8.

if I had just been given a little more time and encouragement, I could have birthed him without the need for a cesarean section.

When I looked up at Sole Woman, I knew she had run over her scheduled hour with me, and she whispered, "Don't worry, don't get up too fast, you have plenty of time." At that moment, I felt so grateful to have this kind, wise woman in my life. Sole Woman suggested that for that day, I take the day off, go to a body of water, the beach, and just sit, rest, relax, trust, and let go. To finish writing my book, I realized that I needed another attentive woman who would give me gentle, firm encouragement along with physical support. I needed this additional labor assistant.

Just as there is no perfect way to give birth, there is no perfect way to write a book. I suggest to a laboring woman, trust, sit, be in water, just be. This is the same gentle suggestion that was given to me to be able to finish writing this book, to put my story, and those of some of the women who have reached out to me, into the world. I needed, but did not know about, the professional labor support of a woman during the birth of my first child. When women experiencing the most difficult part of their labor are afraid, they need to be told they are strong, and encouraged to trust that they can give birth. Nurturing women and men in their paths will tell them they can do it, that they have the physical and inner strength to give birth naturally to their babies. I cherish the many caring and inspirational individuals in my life. This circle of support helped me give birth to this book.

Chapter 2

Pregnancy and Childbirth
in Women's Psychological Development

In response to our question, "What was the most important learning experience you have ever had?" many mothers selected childbirth. It is as if this act of creation ushers in a whole new view of one's creative capacities.

Mary Field Belenky, Blythe McVicker Clinchy,
Nancy Rule Goldberger, and Jill Mattuck Tarule
Women's Ways of Knowing:
The Development of Self, Voice, and Mind
1986, p. 35

Childbirth represents a major developmental rite of passage in a woman's life. The experience of giving birth and becoming a mother affects every aspect of her existence. With the birth of a woman's first child, she begins a relationship with a new being who is totally dependent on her. Her entire identity is transformed. Childbirth is a pivotal experience that deserves a place of honor in a woman's life and in society.

As a mother, a woman enters a new phase of life, experiences changes in her former relationships, and begins new relationships. With her first child she undertakes a new role of mother, a role that is redefined and extended with each subsequent child. Other social connections—wife, partner, daughter, daughter-in-law, sister, even friend or co-worker—are likely to be considerably changed by her becoming a mother. Psychological models of women's development affirm that this stage of a woman's life needs to be viewed in the context of the creation of new and changing relationships.

Jean Baker Miller's *Toward a New Psychology of Women* (1976) was a groundbreaking book that defined women's psychological development as different from traditional male-oriented developmental theory. Miller and other feminist scholars affiliated with the Stone Center for Developmental Services and Studies at Wellesley College state that, for women, relationships define developmental stages (Jordan et al., 1991). Whereas the Eriksonian developmental model centers on "separation-individuation," in which increasing independence and self-sufficiency define health and maturity, the Stone Center model focuses on women's growth through connection with others. Its basic premise is ". . . for women at all life stages, relational needs are primary and that healthy, dynamic relationships are the motivating force that propels psychological growth" (Surrey in Jordan, Surrey, and Kaplan, 1991, p. 37).

According to Miller, "The very essence of all life is growth, which means change. The one great additional feature that characterizes human growth is psychological change. . . . Change and growth are intimate parts of women's lives" (1976, pp. 55-57). A special opportunity for change and growth exists for women during pregnancy, childbirth, and postpartum.

Ellen Galinsky, lecturer on child and adult development, describes six stages that expectant parents experience. The nurturing stage takes place during the birth of the baby. She writes,

> The major task of this stage is to form an attachment to the baby . . . . Accepting their new role, parents have to enlarge their relationships to each other, their other children (if they have them), and their own parents to include the baby, to redefine these relationships, and then to try to right the imbalance created by the birth, particularly to their sense of self. . . . Part of the task of forming the attachment to the new baby is reconciling the actual birth with the imagined birth. (Galinsky, 1981, pp. 48-49)

In my work, the reconciling to which Galinsky refers occurs in the telling of the birth story. It is for this reason that I encourage women to share and listen to birth stories while preparing for an upcoming birth. In postpartum sessions, this practice helps the woman to go on to the job of mothering.

In *Special Women: The Role of the Professional Labor Assistant* (Perez and Snedeker, 1990), Polly Perez, professional labor assistant, perinatal nurse, childbirth educator, and hospital consultant defines three emotional stages of pregnancy that coincide with the three trimesters: incorporation, differentiation, and separation.

Perez sees the first trimester as a common time of ambivalence about the pregnancy and motherhood. Pregnant women need to be reassured by their caregivers that these feelings are normal. The task of this stage is acceptance of the pregnancy and incorporation of this new image of the self. Perez suggests that, during the first trimester, women need support from their health care providers in dealing with the physical changes they experience. Guidance with appropriate nutrition and exercise is beneficial. It is important for a woman to feel that her body is strong enough to give birth.

The second trimester is a period of differentiation, during which the pregnant woman sees her developing baby as a being separate from herself. "She begins to think of herself as a mother and may spend much time talking to her own mother" (Perez and Snedeker, 1990, p. 72). By this time, the woman should no longer be conflicted about the pregnancy. Perez notes that, "Uterine dystocia in labor is very common if there are unresolved ambivalent feelings after the fifth month of pregnancy" (p. 72).

The third trimester is the time when the pregnant woman begins the work of separation from the baby growing inside of her. The woman looks inward and begins to see the baby as a real child. She prepares for the birth by taking childbirth classes and begins to trust in her body's ability to give birth. She continues to need to feel supported by those around her. Perez concludes that, if these emotional stages are not completed, labor may be slow to progress, and the woman may have difficulty in her transition to her role as a mother.

The period from pregnancy through postpartum presents a unique opportunity for women to grow in all aspects of their lives. The need for women to have special nurturing relationships during this time is consistent with the focus of the Stone Center model of women's development. I have discovered in my work that all women need and benefit from the support of a circle of caring women as they become mothers.

PART II:
BIRTH AS A MEDICAL
INTERVENTION

Chapter 3

Contemporary
Medical Interventions

*Some obstetricians believe that whenever a machine or a proce-
dure is available which permits greater medical control of childbirth, it ought to be used. An equally valid view is that one should
be selective in the use of technology, employing it where necessary, but bearing in mind that birth is also a psychological experience which affects the relationship between mother, father, and
baby—perhaps for a long time after.*

Sheila Kitzinger
*The Complete Book of Pregnancy
and Childbirth*
1996, p. 315

The act of birthing a baby has not changed over time. Yet the
normal, healthy birthing process is given little attention in the medical
school curriculum. Medical staff are trained to deliver the baby, and
attend to any perceived clinical problem during that process. They
receive extensive training in the use of technology in labor (Korte,
1997; Northrup, 1994). This is undoubtedly essential for dealing with
emergency situations, but the widespread medicalization of childbirth,
especially the routine use of technology and pharmacology, often dramatically, negatively, and unnecessarily affects a woman's experience
of giving birth.

BACKGROUND

Until the early 1900s, midwives were the main health care providers
of birthing women in America (Chester, 1997). Around this time,

physicians, all male, began to compete with midwives for patients. Even poor women and immigrants were considered desirable as patients. Eventually the physicians organized into professional groups that enabled them to gain and maintain power over the midwifery community.

In 1920, at the forty-fifth Annual Meeting of the American Gynecological Society, obstetrician Dr. Joseph DeLee presented his views on the need for increased medical intervention in childbirth in an article titled "The Prophylactic Forceps Operation" (DeLee, 1920). This article, promoting the obstetrical management of birth, made such procedures as forceps extraction, episiotomies, and the lithotomy position standard practice. The lithotomy position requires the woman to lie in bed flat on her back with her legs in stirrups, forcing the baby to be pushed or pulled upward because of the consequent curve of the birth canal. DeLee advocated that women be sedated through labor and made unconscious for delivery. He described birth as a very dangerous event for women and babies, an "operation" performed by a surgeon on a patient to save the mother and baby. Dr. DeLee's campaign to abolish midwives succeeded because his theory of childbirth as a life-threatening medical/surgical event to be managed by physicians rather than midwives was accepted as fact, forcing an end to midwifery as the primary agency of childbirth (Litoff, 1978, p. 67). By the 1930s, midwifery came to an end as a respected profession in this country, and childbirth occurred primarily in hospitals (Rothman, 1991; Chester, 1997).

From the 1920s to the present time, many changes have occurred in the way that women give birth in the United States. The women's liberation movement of the 1970s had a profound impact on childbirth. The book, *Our Bodies, Ourselves: A Book By and For Women,* first published in 1970 (The Boston Women's Health Book Collective, Inc.), became an important guide for women seeking control of their health care, including their pregnancies and births. Women and their partners began to advocate for natural childbirth and more involvement by men in the birthing process. Couples took childbirth preparation classes to ready themselves for the birth of their babies. Men began attending the births of their children. By the late 1980s, in response to the natural childbirth movement, hospitals began to offer the option of low-risk women delivering in birthing centers rather than the delivery room. In the 1990s, pregnant women and their partners benefit greatly from these changes and the choices available to them. However, widespread use of medical interventions still exists.

COMMON
MEDICAL INTERVENTIONS

Many of the medical interventions in childbirth instituted in the United States in the 1920s continue to be common practice in today's hospitals. These and many other interventions introduced since then are routine, ostensibly as a means of improving the care of women giving birth and their babies. There are certainly situations in which medical technology is necessary and important to the health of the mother and the baby. But the standard use of these interventions has limited benefits for low-risk women and their babies, and they carry many potential disadvantages. Research has identified a number of problems that can result from the medical management of childbirth. For example, each intervention that is introduced is likely to lead to another one. This issue is a major reason for the great number of cesarean sections (Cohen and Estner, 1983). It does not appear that many of the medical controls used in most hospitals produce healthier babies and mothers (Klaus, Kennell, and Klaus, 1993).

Pitocin

Time is an important consideration when childbirth is seen as a medical event. A woman enters the hospital in labor and the medical staff begin to count the time as it elapses. Her bed may be perceived as being needed by another laboring "patient." Many physicians believe that a woman should labor and give birth within a set time period. Doctors who think of a particular labor as "slow" may therefore prescribe a drug, Pitocin, to speed up the labor.

Pitocin brings on contractions artificially and causes contractions to increase in intensity and frequency. These contractions are much more uncomfortable than natural contractions that are experienced without the administration of the drug. Because these induced contractions are quite painful, the use of Pitocin often leads to other medical interventions such as pain medication or epidural anesthesia, an anesthetic given to the laboring woman to relieve the pain. Epidural anesthesia presents other risks during labor.

The time pressure is exacerbated by strict adherence to the "Friedman labor curve." This curve represents the average dilation for a laboring woman as one centimeter per hour in the active stage of labor. Many practitioners follow this curve as a strict rule, rather than the average measure of progress. Its originator, Dr. Emanuel Friedman, a professor of obstetrics and gynecology at Harvard Medical School, has asserted that "the Friedman labor curve is being abused more than it is being used appropriately and that to intervene with a cesarean for prolonged labor is unthinkable" (Young, 1987, p. 13). The conclusion that labor is progressing too slowly is often made because the woman enters the hospital and starts the time clock earlier than is necessary.

In certain situations women may feel satisfied with Pitocin as a medical intervention that helped them give birth. If women were allowed to labor without time pressure, however, it is possible that the use of Pitocin could be decreased.

Prescribed Fasting

In many hospitals, a woman under the care of an obstetrician is not allowed to eat or drink while in labor. "The purpose of fasting is to prevent the aspiration of stomach contents under (general) anesthesia, *should* anesthesia become necessary" (Herzfeld, 1985, p. 26). This practice is often interrelated with other medical interventions.

Once a woman has been in the hospital for a number of hours without food or drink she will tend to become dehydrated, in which case intravenous fluids will be prescribed. Hooked up to an IV, a woman finds it more difficult to walk around comfortably. Her self-perception may change significantly. Prior to the IV she is a pregnant woman but not a sick woman. Many women have shared with me their feelings of not having any control over their bodies after being started on the IV. They feel they are no longer healthy; they feel they need to be taken care of by the medical staff. Women who stay home during most of labor are less likely to need an IV. If the doctor controls the woman's option to ingest nourishment, she may come to feel that she loses control over making other decisions.

Fasting results in the laboring woman becoming more tired and less able to cope with the difficult, painful task of giving birth. In the event that a nonemergency cesarean section is indicated, a woman is given epidural or spinal anesthesia for the surgery. It is not necessary for a woman to have an empty stomach for these types of anesthesia to be administered. By controlling the patient's intake of food and drink, however, the care provider knows that she has been abstinent while in the hospital and could quickly be prepared for emergency surgery under general anesthesia if necessary.

Emergency cesareans are performed when it is determined that the baby's or mother's health is at significant risk. If the placenta is detaching from the lining of the uterus, for example, severe bleeding occurs and an emergency cesarean is indicated for the mother's safety. With an emergency cesarean, general anesthesia is administered. As in the case of any other emergency surgery, a patient is intubated as a preventive measure whether food has been taken or not. This is common medical practice for emergency surgery, but not a reason to prohibit all laboring women from eating and drinking (Cohen and Estner, 1983).

Laboring women who have continued eating and drinking according to their needs are generally more able to endure long, hard hours of labor without pain-killing drugs and other medical interventions. Light foods such as soup, eggs, or yogurt, eaten during early labor, help to fortify the woman for the often difficult and long process of laboring and giving birth.

Electronic Fetal Monitoring

The external electronic fetal monitor was originally introduced in the 1970s for high-risk pregnancies such as multiple births, or for diabetic or toxemic patients. The monitor has become a standard piece of equipment in American hospital labor rooms. External fetal monitoring is the continuous monitoring of the baby's heartbeat by a transducer placed on the woman's abdomen. It is routine practice in many hospitals for a laboring woman upon admission to be attached to the external fetal monitor to have a twenty- to thirty-minute assessment of the baby's heart rate. The woman must stay in bed for the monitor to pick up the fetal heart tones and measure the contractions. Most women feel uncomfortable staying in bed during labor and say they are more comfortable if they are able to walk around between contractions. No studies of low-risk women have shown any benefits from the use of fetal monitoring (Flamm, 1990; Kitzinger, 1996). Although electronic fetal monitoring was believed to make childbirth safer for babies, studies have shown that it does not.

The necessity of a cesarean cannot be based solely on the electronic fetal monitor readout. Sometimes the monitor registers that the baby is "in distress," and simply moving the woman into an upright position will stabilize the baby's heartbeat. Without the monitor the woman would probably not be on her back in labor, especially if there are any signs of fetal distress.

Dr. Edward Hon, inventor of the electronic fetal monitor (EFM), cautioned other physicians about its use. He commented that "Not all patients should be electronically monitored. Most women in labor are much better off at home than in the hospital with the electronic fetal monitor. . . . We've forgotten that most women deliver in time. If you allow twenty-four hours to elapse before intervening, you wouldn't have the high cesarean rate" (Young, 1987, p. 14).

Between 1970 and 1978, while the fetal monitor was being introduced, the diagnosis of dystocia, or "failure to progress," doubled in this country (Korte and Scaer, 1984, p. 146). In the late 1990s approximately one-third of cesareans are performed for dystocia (Korte, 1997). Electronic fetal monitoring increases the cesarean section rate by 160 percent (Kitzinger, 1996).

Since this technology provides "privileged" information, the doctors and nurses are assumed to understand what the machinery means, while the laboring woman and those supporting her do not (Jordan, 1987, p. 38). It is not uncommon for medical staff to interpret normal variations in the fetal heartbeat as pathological. "Half of all babies show there are some irregularities of heartbeat during labor. Usually this is of no significance" (Kitzinger, 1996, p. 333). It is Kitzinger's opinion that incomplete understanding of the normal range of the fetal heartbeat leads to a great deal of intervention and unnecessary increase in cesarean sections.

An alternative to the fetal monitor, the fetoscope, is a type of stethoscope that does not require invasive technology and is designed to hear the fetal heartbeat. The fetoscope effectively measures the fetal heartbeat without interfering with a woman's ability to stay mobile during labor (Kitzinger, 1996; Korte, 1997; Rothman, 1991). The American College of Obstetrics and Gynecology (ACOG) now endorses a policy of continual listening with the ultrasound stethoscope as better than electronic fetal monitoring. Unfortunately, most care providers have not been trained to provide this service and they continue to utilize electronic fetal monitoring (Kitzinger, 1996).

Epidural Anesthesia

Epidural anesthesia, an anesthetic that is injected into the spine, numbing the woman from the waist to the toes, is given to alleviate the pain of labor. Epidural is the most popular labor medication in the United States, used in some hospitals on 90 percent of the women in labor (Korte, 1997). For many women, labor is perceived as an intolerable pain that they do not wish to endure. Although it is widely used, epidural anesthesia may carry a risk to the baby, because like other drugs used in labor, it crosses the placenta and enters the baby's bloodstream (Korte, 1997, p. 153). Possible problems associated with epidural anesthesia include arrest of the labor, fever, increased forceps use, pelvic floor damage, and fetal distress (Northrup, 1994).

Epidural anesthesia has also been related to increased cesarean section rates (Kennell et al., 1991; Klaus, Kennell, and Klaus, 1993; Korte, 1997; Northrup, 1994). Because a woman is anesthetized, she is not able to assume an upright position in order to more efficiently push her baby out. In addition, epidural anesthesia itself may slow down the labor by changing the strength and frequency of contractions so that they are less effective. Epidural anesthesia also may cause a drop in the mother's blood pressure, another condition that could have serious consequences for her or her baby (Korte, 1997).

Episiotomy

Episiotomy, the most common obstetric operation, is the only surgical procedure performed on a healthy woman without her consent (Crawford and Walters, 1996). It is a surgical cut of the vagina made to enlarge the birth opening. It is performed under local anesthesia just before the birth, presumably to prevent vaginal tearing or to allow for a quicker delivery in cases of fetal distress. Though not indicated in the majority of births, it is still routinely taught in OB/GYN residency programs (Northrup, 1994). Currently, as women have begun to question the need for routine episiotomy, obstetricians are also asking about its extensive use (Kitzinger, 1996). Although most women do not feel the episiotomy when it is made, it can be painful and susceptible to infection for weeks and even months afterward. Approximately 65 percent of women giving birth in the United States receive an episiotomy (Korte, 1997). In some hospitals, almost 100 percent of women undergo this surgical procedure (Northrup, 1994, p. 393).

Anecdotally, when asked about episiotomy, most of my prenatal and postpartum clients report that they trusted their physician would make the correct decision about the necessity of an episiotomy. Those who had an episiotomy were surprised to learn that it was in fact a standard surgical procedure, not generally based on case-by-case need. They stated that the episiotomy was a painful experience, but felt that the decision to perform the procedure must have been warranted. After finding out this might not have been true, however, there were three common themes in their responses.

The most commonly held position was implicit trust in a physician to make the best decision about an episiotomy for the health of the baby. A second theme emerged when I suggested discussing the procedure with their care providers: many women did not want to "bother" the physician with questions because he or she was seen as an important person who knew what was best for the woman. A small number of women held a third view, which was one of anger and resentment. These women were shocked and surprised that this painful surgical procedure was in fact optional, only indicated when the baby is at risk. Kitzinger writes, "As soon as a research project investigating episiotomy was begun in any hospital—that is, as soon as questions were raised about its necessity—the rate dropped by about a third, even before any results were obtained" (1996, p. 322).

Many women have come to expect that technology will aid them in giving birth. Rather, studies have shown that medical interventions do not necessarily improve birth outcome and, in fact, may detract from the birth experience of the mother (Kitzinger, 1996). Women whose pregnancies are proceeding normally need more support, not more medical management.

Chapter 4

The Cesarean Section

A common saying among obstetricians is, "The only cesarean I've ever been sued for is the one I didn't do." It is unfortunate but true that until something can be done about misguided lawsuits, the cesarean section rate is not likely to fall.

Bruce L. Flamm
Birth After Cesarean
1990, p. 23

One major problem that has resulted from the medical management of childbirth is the high rate of cesarean section. Cesarean section is the most commonly performed operation in the United States (Cohen and Estner, 1983; Crawford and Walters, 1996; Flamm, 1990; Myers and Gleicher, 1988; Stafford, 1990). The frequency of this surgery has increased dramatically during the past thirty years. In 1970, 5.5 percent of all hospital births were cesarean sections and by the mid-1980s 24 percent of all births were by cesarean. The rate hovers at approximately 24 percent in the 1990s (Crawford and Walters, 1996; Kitzinger, 1996)—this in spite of the trend toward "natural childbirth." There has not been an increase in the newborn survival rate with the current high rate of cesarean. In Britain the cesarean section rate is about 15 percent, and in the Netherlands it is less than 10 percent (Kitzinger, 1996).

Cesarean section can be a lifesaving surgery, and out of necessity cesarean sections will always be performed. Some conditions, though they occur rarely, are clear indications for cesarean: prolapsed umbilical cord, placenta previa, placental abruption, and an active outbreak of herpes at the time of birth. Prolapsed cord is a situation in which the cord descends through the cervix before the baby does. The baby may pinch the cord and drastically reduce its oxygen supply, necessitating immediate cesarean section. Placenta previa occurs when the placenta covers or partially covers the cervix. As the cervix dilates, the placenta separates from the uterus, causing painless bleeding in the mother and depriving the fetus of oxygen. The incidence of placenta previa is about one in every two hundred births (Korte, 1997). Placental abruption occurs when the placenta prematurely separates from the uterine wall. This may cause vaginal bleeding and, if a significant amount of the placenta has come away, often necessitates a cesarean. The cause of placental abruption is unknown, but the condition may be associated with malnutrition and high blood pressure. In the case of herpes, if there is a herpes lesion at the time of the birth, most health care providers opt for cesarean section to protect the baby from infection with the herpes virus. Herpes can have serious health consequences in the newborn.

Physicians perform cesareans for other reasons, including dystocia, fetal distress, and breech presentation (Stafford, 1990). There is considerable controversy about cesareans being done for these reasons. The uses of medical interventions such as epidural anesthesia and electronic fetal monitoring may also lead to unnecessary cesareans.

Dystocia, prolonged or difficult labor, is a controversial and yet common justification for cesareans. Another diagnosis for a cesarean due to long labor is "failure to progress." There may be difficulty in the progress of the labor for any of three reasons: weak contractions ("uterine inertia"); a poor position of the fetus; or an abnormal-sized pelvis (cephalopelvic disproportion—CPD) that prevents the baby from descending through the mother's birth canal (Korte, 1997).

According to the literature, and in my experience with women in labor, many women have long labors that are normal and not dangerous for them or the baby. Cesarean sections are frequently performed because a woman simply becomes depleted of energy as she is going through a long labor. This diagnosis cannot be reliably made until the active phase of labor, after five centimeters dilation, since the early phase of labor, zero to four centimeters, is often very slow (Simkin, Whalley, and Keppler, 1991). In my work, I suggest that women stay home with supportive people until they are in the active stage of labor. Part of the problem with the diagnosis of dystocia lies in the fact that many women go to the hospital too early in the labor and the medical staff begin timing "progress" on admission.

Uterine dystocia is very common during labor. We do not know why women's labors often slow down at five or six centimeters dilation. Sometimes a woman's body simply needs a rest from labor, so the labor slows down. A woman's labor may slow down when she enters the hospital because of the change from laboring in the home with people she knows and trusts.

Many women are told by their physicians that their pelvis size is "too small" to birth a baby vaginally and they need a cesarean section. The pelvis is a bony structure that has ligaments attached to it that become flexible toward the end of pregnancy and during labor. By assuming an upright position for labor, and especially a squatting position for the pushing stage, a woman can usually push her baby out; her body is just the right size to give birth in this posture. Rarely, a woman will have a truly contracted pelvis, due to polio or a childhood fracture, and she needs a cesarean (Flamm, 1990).

Many women who have a cesarean because of a diagnosis of CPD or "too small for a vaginal birth," subsequently give birth to a larger baby than the cesarean baby (Cohen and Estner, 1983; Korte, 1997). My experience confirms this; of the women I have worked with, most have given birth vaginally to a larger baby after a cesarean that had been performed for CPD. Two women in a VBAC class a few years ago had been told that they were too small to have vaginal births. They had had cesareans for six- and seven-pound babies. During their subsequent pregnancies, we discussed this issue in the group setting among other couples. These couples expressed a great deal of anger at being told that the women were too small to give birth vaginally. I remember the joy expressed by both of these mothers when they told me of their VBAC babies, both born weighing over nine pounds.

At the end of gestation, 3 to 4 percent of babies are in the breech position and 80 percent of these are born by cesarean section. It is possible for a trained obstetrician to deliver a breech baby vaginally with little risk of complications (Kitzinger, 1996). The reason for the high rate of cesarean for breech babies is that few American obstetricians are trained to deliver a breech baby vaginally. In recent years,

American medical students have not been trained to deliver breech babies vaginally (Cohen, 1991; Korte, 1997).

Age is another factor in a doctor's decision to perform a cesarean section. The rate of cesarean section increases with a woman's age. In 1994 when the overall cesarean rate was 22 percent in this country, the cesarean rate was 24.2 percent for women ages 30 to 34, 27.7 percent for women ages 35 to 39, and 31.5 percent for women age 40 and older (Korte, 1997, p. 57). Each woman should be individually assessed, based on her health status and other relevant factors. One of my goals is to educate women and their partners about potential medical interventions during labor and childbirth so that they can make informed choices about their use, and to assist women who have had a previous cesarean to maximize their chances of a safe vaginal birth of future babies.

"ONCE A CESAREAN, ALWAYS A CESAREAN":
A DISCUSSION

In 1916, Dr. Edwin Cragin wrote an article for the *New York Medical Journal* stating that cesarean section, because of its danger to the mother, should not be performed unless it was absolutely necessary. His phrase, "Once a cesarean, always a cesarean" was spoken in reference to the danger of repeating a cesarean at that time in medical history (Cragin, 1916). In the past, women with previous cesareans were routinely subjected to repeat cesareans because of fear of uterine rupture during subsequent labor (Clark, 1988; Crawford and Walters, 1996; Flamm, 1990). At the time of Dr. Cragin's article, cesareans were dangerous because most of them were performed using a "classical" incision, a vertical incision on the uterus that weakened it in subsequent hard contractions of labor, making uterine rupture a serious threat to a woman's life. Today the risk of uterine rupture is very low since 90 percent of cesareans are performed using a low transverse incision, making vaginal birth after cesarean safe in most cases after this type of cesarean section (Flamm, 1990). A low transverse incision, which is a horizontal incision on the uterus, is less damaging to the uterus and "the chances of a woman dying during VBAC are infinitesimal, regardless of the kind of incision on the uterus. In contrast, women die every year from complications of scheduled repeat cesarean, not related to the uterine scar at all but simply because cesarean is major abdominal surgery with all its attendant risks" (Crawford and Walters, 1996, p. 33).

Fear of maternal death from uterine rupture was the primary reason for physicians' reluctance to accept the feasibility of vaginal birth after cesarean. In a 1990 review of forty-three medical articles published over the previous thirty-five years, of the 11,027 women in the studies who attempted vaginal birth after cesarean, no woman died due to uterine rupture (Flamm, 1990, p. 30). In addition, each of these reports supports the safety of vaginal birth after cesarean (p. 63). Other studies arrived at the same conclusion. "The low transverse uterine incision is considered by the medical community to have such a low risk of rupture that a woman with this uterine incision is in the same category as a woman who has never had uterine surgery" (Crawford and Walters, 1996, p. 31).

Nevertheless, previous cesareans accounted for 48 percent of the increase in cesareans from 1980 through 1985 (Taffel, Placek, and Liss, 1987). "Many obstetricians feel inherently that vaginal delivery is just plain dangerous, leading to increased fetal trauma" (Northrup, 1994, p. 392). This fear of danger to the baby is another reason for the many unnecessary cesareans.

The National Institutes of Health's report of its Task Force to Lower the Cesarean Rate, published in 1980, advocated specific goals to lower the cesarean section rate. Its findings included modifying the statement, "Once a cesarean, always a cesarean"; breech delivery should no longer be an acceptable reason for cesarean; the diagnosis of fetal distress needed improved exactness; and dystocia was diagnosed too often (Petitti, 1985, p. 25). Unfortunately the recommendations did not improve the national patterns of practice. Despite its demonstrated safety, VBAC attempts are still not encouraged by many physicians. Nine out of ten cesarean women still undergo elective repeat cesarean on the advice of their physicians (Flamm, 1990).

In 1982, ACOG announced a policy change of not advocating repeat cesarean sections for women who have had one or more cesareans. They concluded that vaginal birth is safer for the woman and the baby than repeat cesarean. Unfortunately, this change did not seem to affect obstetrical practice to any large degree. Many doctors may feel more comfortable following familiar practices. Women who have been frightened by a physician's comments about uterine rupture may be relieved to agree to the cesarean unquestioningly. In a 1996 editorial in *The New England Journal of Medicine,* Dr. Richard Paul advises an attempt of labor with the objective of vaginal birth for women who have had a previous cesarean as a critical means of reducing the number of elective cesareans, stating, "Although 'once a cesarean, always a scar' is a truism, it is not true that once a cesarean, always a cesarean" (Paul, 1996, p. 736).

REDUCING THE CESAREAN RATE

Statistics show that as many as one quarter of all babies in the United States and Canada are born by cesarean section, and that about half of these are performed because the mother had a previous cesarean (McMahon et al., 1996). The rate of cesarean section could be lowered drastically without adverse effects on the health of babies (Flamm, 1990; Korte, 1997). Simkin, Whalley, and Kepler (1991) contend, based on research in the medical literature, that the cesarean rate can safely be lowered to 12 to 15 percent. The World Health Organization suggested the cesarean section rate should be lowered to 10 to 12 percent or lower (Kitzinger, 1996). Other studies have shown that the rate could be even lower (Porreco, 1985; Myers and Gleicher, 1988).

For women who have undergone cesarean section, it must be acknowledged that having a baby and major abdominal surgery at the same time may result in significant medical and emotional consequences. There are multiple reasons, both physical and psychological, that the rate of cesarean section should be lowered. Potential medical risks to the mother include blood loss, blood clots, and infection of the uterus, urinary tract, and the surgical wound (Crawford and Walters, 1996, pp. 28-29). Cesarean section may affect a woman's ability to have a rewarding birth experience as well as a positive immediate postbirth bonding experience with her baby. Many women who have cesarean births are filled with sadness after the disappointment of not having a vaginal birth. They may withdraw, feel angry, or experience denial, self-blame, guilt, or depression. As the cesarean mother recovers physically and adjusts to her new baby, intense feelings or memories of the experience may begin to surface. She may question her image of herself as a woman.

Myers and Gleicher (1988) developed an initiative to decrease the cesarean rate in an inner-city hospital. They established a protocol that consisted of requiring a second opinion prior to all cesarean sections, setting standard criteria for the four most common indications for cesarean births (previous cesarean section, dystocia, breech presentation, and fetal distress), and an extensive review of all cesareans and of individual obstetricians' rates of performing them. Attending physicians' participation in the program was voluntary. The authors report that the overall cesarean rate was reduced from 17.5 percent to 11 percent during the first two years of the study. Only the decrease in the primary cesarean rate, from 12 to 6.8 percent, was statistically significant. The study shows that this type of program can significantly reduce cesarean section rates without harmful effects on the mother or baby.

Another study was undertaken at St. Luke's Hospital in Denver, Colorado, in which several cesarean reduction strategies were instituted for the clinic births. Residents attended the births and the hospital lowered the cesarean rate for the clinic mothers from 17.6 to 5.7 percent. St. Luke's did not attempt to introduce the same policy on the private service, where the cesarean rate remained at 17.6 percent (Porreco, 1985).

Winthrop Hospital's (Long Island, New York) cesarean rate was 30 percent when Dr. Harold Schulman, chief of OB/GYN, instituted a policy of peer review for all cesareans and active encouragement of a trial of labor for women who had had previous cesareans. Following his program, the rate decreased by 10 percent within a few months (Norwood, 1986).

In 1994, under a program sponsored by Massachusetts Blue Cross/ Blue Shield, ten Massachusetts hospitals began a program to reduce their rates of cesarean sections. A number of strategies were employed, including deferring admission into the hospital until the labor had significantly progressed, delaying the use of epidural anesthesia, decreasing routine electronic fetal monitoring, encouraging walking during labor, and not assigning a specific due date for the birth. These efforts reduced the collective cesarean rate in these hospitals from 25 percent in 1994 to 20 percent in 1997. By September 1998, forty-one hospitals in Massachusetts were involved in this program; only ten of the state's obstetrical units did not participate. Through the Boston-based Institute for Healthcare Improvement, fifty-six hospitals, health plans, and provider networks throughout the country have joined this effort to reduce cesarean rates. According to participants in this program, "This translates into hundreds fewer surgical births with no compromise in good outcomes" (Knox, 1998, p. C4).

An additional important step to reduce the rate of cesarean section is to communicate information concerning its potential dangers to consumers. Childbirth educators can be among those who prevent unnecessary cesareans by informing clients of their options. They have the opportunity to inform women of the benefits of believing in their bodies' abilities to give birth.

POSTPARTUM EFFECTS

Some women feel satisfied and content with having their babies by cesarean section. For many others, however, a cesarean has profound physical and psychological effects. The mother is not only affected by the stress of surgical birth and the recovery time needed, she is often left with an emotional scar from which she needs to recover. It is important for a woman to know that she may experience feelings of loss if she has a cesarean section.

Most women do not acknowledge their grief after a cesarean until some time has elapsed during which they can process the birth experience. Women often tell me they feel guilty about experiencing sadness after a cesarean section. They expect that they ought to be happy and satisfied if they have a healthy baby. I respond that a feeling of satisfaction for a healthy baby is appropriate, but sadness and grief are also natural emotions following the surgical birth of a baby.

With a cesarean, the mother usually does not see the baby until she is out of the recovery room, many hours after the birth. This may affect the new mother on many levels. She may worry about the newborn when she cannot physically see her or him; nursing the infant is delayed; and she loses the very important contact with the newborn during the first hours of life.

A study of vaginal and cesarean deliveries compared the length of time between birth and when the baby was first held by the mother. Of the vaginal birth mothers, 44 percent held the baby immediately after the birth, and another 44 percent held the baby within the first hour after birth. Of the women who gave birth by cesarean, 9 percent held the baby within two hours of the birth and another 9 percent held the baby between two and four hours after the birth. The remaining 82 percent held the baby for the first time six or more hours after birth (Bradley, Ross, and Warnyca, 1983).

In another study of women three to six days postpartum, the mother-infant contact also occurred significantly later in the cesarean group than in the vaginal birth group. In the cesarean group, 22 percent of the women could not remember precisely the moment of first contact. When asked about their enjoyment of the baby, the cesarean group replied significantly more frequently than the vaginal birth group that they were "having too much pain to enjoy the baby." The moment the women fed their infants for the first time was also considerably delayed in the cesarean group (Garel, Lelong, and Kaminski, 1987, p. 203).

When women tell me that they did not hold their babies for a few hours after birth, or even for as much as twenty-four hours after their cesarean section, they express grief and feelings of loss about this. Sometimes women feel unsure whether the baby is definitely theirs and may experience guilt over their doubts. Some say they had not cared about holding the baby because they had felt so physically uncomfortable. Many women stated that they grieved over the memory of not seeing their babies and not caring about seeing them. This indicates the importance of the emotional need for mothers and their newborns to have physical contact soon after a cesarean section.

The cesarean group in another study tended to view their births as not normal. Satisfaction with their birth experience was significantly lower among cesarean women. The findings of this study suggested that a cesarean section delivery has a negative impact on the woman's understanding of her labor and childbirth experience. The psychological and emotional stresses in the cesarean group included feelings of loss of control, fear, guilt, anxiety, and failure (Marut and Mercer, 1979).

Unlike other abdominal surgeries planned in advance, a primary cesarean generally occurs without forewarning and without preparation for a period of convalescence. Pain, exhaustion, depression, and anger are therefore likely to follow and the family and doctor who counsels the couple need to be aware of these reactions. (Debrovner and Shubin, 1985, p. 90)

Women's satisfaction in the early postpartum period is negatively affected by a cesarean. In one study, women who were contacted within twenty-four to forty-eight hours of giving birth were assessed for satisfaction with the delivery after an emergency cesarean and after a vaginal birth. The emergency cesarean group reported considerably less satisfaction with their childbirth experiences than did women in the vaginal birth group (Padawer et al., 1988).

When comparing a cesarean group and a group of women who delivered vaginally in another study, the cesarean group was found to have a higher number of obstetrical complications, a greater rate of depression, and a lengthier recovery period. There was substantially more depression during the first month postpartum among cesarean women than among women who experienced vaginal birth. Feelings of failure and lowered self-esteem were present for the cesarean mother (Gottlieb and Barrett, 1986).

According to another study, women who had given birth by cesarean were more likely to make more medical visits during the first year than the women who had birthed vaginally. The main symptoms reported by cesarean mothers were depression, sleep problems, and headaches. They felt less confident in their ability to care for their babies (Garel, Lelong, and Kaminski, 1988).

In my practice I find a woman may experience emotions of sadness as the baby grows out of infancy and she begins to have some time to herself. It is also very common for a woman to start experiencing her grief when she is pregnant again.

Currently cesarean sections account for approximately 25 percent of all births in the United States. This means that a significant percentage of women are recuperating from major abdominal surgery while adapting to the challenges and wonders of motherhood, a major life transition. Women need to be reassured that grief is a natural and expected part of their recovery from a cesarean section. They also deserve to be educated about preventing unnecessary cesareans.

PART III:
BIRTH AS AN EXPERIENCE
OF EMPOWERMENT

Chapter 5

Support for Honoring
the Experience of Childbirth

When enough women realize that birth is a time of great opportunity to get in touch with their true power, and when they are willing to assume responsibility for this, we will reclaim the power of birth and help move technology where it belongs—in the service of birthing women, not as their master.

Christiane Northrup
Women's Bodies, Women's Wisdom
1994, p. 413

Giving birth can be an empowering experience in a woman's life because she and her partner have the opportunity to make important choices that influence the outcome of this significant life event. They are able to research and select the childbirth educator, health care providers, and the people who will support them during and after pregnancy. Couples become confident by gaining information and working for the birth experience they want for themselves. A woman needs encouragement to look to her inner resources and discover ways that she can take care of herself during pregnancy. She has many of her own answers. Choosing supportive people and utilizing the following suggestions during childbirth preparation helps the woman and her partner prepare for the birth.

THE CHILDBIRTH EDUCATOR

The childbirth educator can provide nurturing care to women and their partners during childbirth preparation sessions. The support of an individual who is knowledgeable about pregnancy, birth, and post-partum is invaluable. In many societies this helpful role falls to older female relatives and neighbors, but in our society such people are much less likely to be available. Childbirth educators, midwives, doulas, and care providers are able to fill this need.

Traditional childbirth education classes serve a beneficial purpose in which the educator informs the woman and her partner about the stages of labor and relaxation techniques. In most childbirth classes a great deal of time is spent teaching breathing techniques. The couple is instructed to learn and practice the breathing techniques to facilitate the birth of the baby. This can give women the false impression that knowing how to breathe through contractions will ensure a control-lable labor. In addition to focusing time on breathing techniques, women need to learn and be encouraged that their bodies are strong, and that they can cope with painful contractions.

In my model of childbirth preparation, the educator helps ready and empower the woman for the experience of childbirth by encouraging her to make informed choices about the upcoming birth. My childbirth classes consist of sessions that provide traditional information as well as time to address the emotional issues that arise. We practice relax-ation and visualization exercises that are useful during both pregnancy and labor. I also stress the importance of being well-informed about less familiar options and alternatives. My clients learn that they can make choices by deciding when to arrive at the hospital and who will support them during labor. I talk with them about trusting their bodies and not fearing the physical pain of labor, but actually surrendering to it as a necessary part of the birth process. For the pregnant woman with no serious medical conditions, I present pregnancy as a healthy period in her life.

We discuss choices the pregnant woman can make to take care of herself in addition to the standard recommendations of regular pre-natal visits and good nutrition. Practicing yoga aids in physical fit-ness, relaxation, and breathing. Chiropractic adjustments are helpful for maintaining health. Many forms of body work are available to help ease the physical and emotional aspects of pregnancy. Thera-peutic massage, reflexology, and energy healing such as reiki can provide relief from the bodily stresses of pregnancy while offering much-needed relaxation. The benefits of massage include muscle relaxation and release of physical and emotional tension. Reflexology utilizes pressure points in the feet for therapeutic purposes. Reiki accesses healing through focused touch, providing compassionate care. A pregnant woman can obtain a referral from her care provider for qualified practitioners of these services. These modalities are of great benefit throughout the pregnancy and postpartum period, supplying the woman with special time to be nurtured.

Another decision a healthy woman can make is to remain at home during early labor as long as possible and continue with normal activities such as eating, drinking fluids, walking, and resting. Labor is a natural process and does not need to be treated as an illness. Encouraging a woman to sleep or rest if she is tired and to proceed with normal activities as long as she feels comfortable doing so is of great benefit. Eating light meals and drinking fluids is important for her to maintain her strength during labor. Taking a shower or bath helps a laboring woman relax. Women generally state that they felt less pain when they walked during labor than when they stayed in bed for long periods of time.

In a study to assess whether walking during active labor was beneficial (Bloom et al., 1998), results showed that walking neither enhanced nor impaired active labor and that it was not harmful to the women or the babies. Among the walkers, 99 percent said they would choose to walk again during another labor. The results of this study suggest that whereas walking does not seem to influence medical consequences, it does make a difference to the woman's experience of labor.

In an individual childbirth preparation series, I educate the woman or couple as I would in a group class. With the privacy of individual sessions, I also focus on any issues that either person would like to discuss such as previous miscarriages or other reproductive losses. Some couples prefer this type of preparation so that they can gain specialized attention for their personal situations. Pregnancy and the postpartum period present an important time for processing issues that are present for either member of the couple.

Childbirth educators can serve as a source of support for exploring emotional issues such as fear, stress, or loss. While working with a client, I address the specific issues that she would like to discuss, using the asking of questions as an assessment skill. I encourage her to tell me about herself, her life, asking one or two questions to begin.

How does she feel about being pregnant? Is she working physically hard at her job? How is she sleeping? Does she have a plan for returning to work or staying home after the baby is born? All of these questions open up areas of further discussion for me to be able to best help her prepare for the upcoming birth.

Fear is a common theme for pregnant women. With a first pregnancy, a woman may have anxiety about the bodily changes she is experiencing. A previous traumatic birth may leave a woman with unresolved issues when she becomes pregnant again. A woman may worry about how she will deal with the pain of labor or whether she will need a medical intervention that she prefers to avoid. Often a woman will speak about her anticipation of the pain of contractions. I may ask her what she is afraid of. As we address her anxiety, I pose a question about her feelings of facing the pain of labor. I encourage her to believe that she has the inner strength to confront the discomfort of labor and remind her that she can also rely on the help of her support people. All women need reassurance that their feelings and fears are important to discuss. By sharing emotions, a woman prepares for the surrendering that is necessary during the birth process and finds some relief from her feelings of apprehension.

An individual may express doubts about being a "good enough" mother. She may expect herself to be perfect. I encourage a woman to know and trust that she does not have to be perfect, that she will do the very best that she can. My gentle questioning regarding her becoming a mother may further the discussion about her experience of being mothered, either years ago or currently. I find a woman may want to speak about her relationship with her mother. If so, we proceed.

Because childbirth educators reach women as adults, many of the cultural messages regarding birth are already deeply ingrained. I emphasize that labor pain is not the pain of illness; rather it is necessary pain in order for the baby to be born. Instead of fearing the pain of labor, women and their partners learn the value of the painful, powerful experience of giving birth.

In a group series, a comfortable environment fosters participation by encouraging people to speak when they are ready to do so. Many women in my classes share their feelings about the physical discomforts of pregnancy and labor. While talking about these discomforts, stress, both physical and emotional, emerges as an important issue.

Some women find pregnancy a time of great peace of mind although others find it to be a time of much uneasiness. They may worry about the health of the developing baby. They may be in physical pain and not be able to maintain their prepregnant level of activity. These issues add to their level of stress.

One man in the group may state that he finds the unfamiliarity of labor stressful, that he does not know how to help his partner when she is in pain. I ask if anyone else feels this way. In most groups, participants will speak at this time. The partners often say that knowing they are not the only one with this concern makes them feel better. I explain that they will be helping the laboring woman by giving support and encouragement to her just as they have under other difficult circumstances.

Women can be helped to discover that they have the resources inside themselves to go through labor, whether through breathing, moaning, groaning, or singing. Vocalization helps women cope with the pain of labor. If a woman is grunting and groaning during contractions, she is often offered epidural anesthesia or medication for pain relief. Encouragement to physically voice her pain is an alternative to the numbing effect of these drugs.

I recommend ways for women to take care of themselves and alleviate stress during pregnancy and new motherhood. One way for a woman to practice self-care is to rest during the early weeks of becoming a mother, rather than resuming former activities as soon as she feels strong. A new mother needs to rest and recuperate after giving birth in order for her body to adjust to the physiological changes of postpregnancy, even if she has had a positive birth experience.

It is helpful for women and partners to be told that feelings of isolation and issues of loss of time, energy, and privacy may emerge as the woman takes on the role of caring for a baby who requires her full attention. Joining a postpartum group led by a sensitive childbirth educator may help them feel less lonely and overwhelmed. A new mother feels supported when she learns that others have shared her surprise and frustration at not being able to find the time to take a shower in the morning. If a woman is struggling with the adjustment to breastfeeding, the group leader may be able to help or provide a referral to a breastfeeding counselor. Depending on the sleeping schedule of the baby, feelings of exhaustion may last more than a few weeks. In this circle of women, participants can support each other by sharing their experiences of intense fatigue and other issues that accompany having a new baby. Women feel better knowing they are not alone with these feelings.

When approaching the end of our prenatal sessions, group or individual, I state that though discussing and planning for the birth is important, the process of giving birth is not something that is controllable. Trusting in the process of birthing is very important. Whatever a woman's religious beliefs or lack thereof, she will have to surrender to the power of the childbirth experience and trust that it is not up to her alone. Tremendous strength can be achieved by a woman looking inward and believing that support and assurance can come from accessing a spiritual connection.

I do not know if a woman will tap into a spiritual relationship during her birthing, but, for me, the energy of a woman giving birth affirms that she and her care providers are not alone in the birthing process. Anyone who has ever had the privilege of being present at a birth knows the miracle that happens every time a new baby comes into the world. I believe that there is a power greater than any of us at the birth of every baby. We are led to believe that the medical technology and the care providers bring the baby into the world. The technology only masks the power that is present for the birthing woman and the strength of her own unique process of giving birth.

I invite a woman and her partner who have had their baby in the previous few months to come to one of the classes to speak about their birth and new parenting experiences. The members of the class enjoy the opportunity to hear the couples' stories and to ask them questions. Listening to descriptions of others' birth experiences helps empower and reassure class participants. At the beginning of the following class, I request reactions to the couple's talk. The most common comment is appreciation for hearing the couple's authentic experience. For some, the session may have intensified fear of the upcoming birth of a new baby. I can then explore these issues.

Helping a woman prepare for the experience of giving birth is sacred, precious work. My goal is that the outcome of her preparation for the birth of her baby is her own growth and healing. My hope for a woman is that she be able to feel the power of this amazing endeavor, of giving birth as a natural experience. Those assisting the laboring woman need to provide encouragement: "You are doing fine, this is the awesome power of the birth experience, it can empower you to live your life, feel your strength as a woman in the world." For the most part, our culture has placed limited value on this perspective of the birth experience. A woman must be encouraged to surrender to the painful, intense contractions that bring about the birth of her baby, rather than relying on the medical interventions frequently suggested. More love, compassion, and support are needed for women giving birth.

Arlene and Tom's Story

Arlene and Tom were preparing for the birth of their twins. During the fourth week of the class series, Tom called to tell me Arlene had given birth to the babies the night before, five weeks before her due date. She and the babies were doing fine. After congratulating him, I spoke to Arlene and asked if they would come to a class in the next few months, to speak about their experience. She decided to come to the very next class, when the babies were only five days old! Arlene, her husband, their friend, and the twins stayed for two hours, talking to us about the birth and the adjustments to new parenting. I knew there was nothing I could tell these pregnant women and their partners that could be more encouraging than their experience of listening to, questioning, and watching this new family.

A few years ago, Arlene called me. I had not heard from her in a number of years. She told me she had just found my name and phone number and wanted to call and tell me the twins were doing well at eight years of age. She remembered the class series and wanted me to know how much it had positively affected her life. I have learned to value and respect this type of assurance that my work with women and couples can have an impact on their lives long after the birth itself.

Dorothy's Story

I worked individually with Dorothy, a thirty-six-year-old woman, during her first pregnancy. After her private sessions, she and her husband, Ted, also attended a small childbirth preparation group that I facilitated. Dorothy is a very spiritual woman with a strong belief that her life is being guided by a higher power.

For years Dorothy had consulted doctors for her menstrual problems. Before we met, Dorothy had undergone a surgical procedure and became pregnant the following month. She considered this pregnancy a miracle. At our second visit, Dorothy shared with me some of the details of her relationship with her mother. She said she felt better after discussing this with me.

Dorothy had strong ideas about what she wanted for the upcoming birth. She very much wanted a natural birth. Even though she was very grateful to her male gynecologist for performing the procedure, she knew she did not want a physician attending her birth. Dorothy found a nurse-midwifery practice for her prenatal care. She spoke often with the two midwives during her prenatal visits about her feelings about and desire for a natural childbirth. The midwives were supportive of her needs.

Dorothy was physically uncomfortable during the evening of the last childbirth preparation class. The next morning she called to tell me her water had broken in the middle of the night, but she was not having contractions yet. Dorothy and her husband spoke to the midwife, who asked them to come into the office so she could listen to the baby's heartbeat. The heartbeat was strong and they returned home to wait. We talked about her resting and continuing her normal routine until labor began.

Dorothy was very excited and could not sleep. After twenty-four hours she prayed for rest and for labor to begin. She then was able to sleep for three hours and her labor woke her.

Dorothy and Ted left for the hospital soon after she woke because of bad weather. Ted was afraid of getting caught in a snowstorm. Dorothy was concerned that she was entering the hospital too early in the labor. Once she was admitted, an internal exam was performed to determine her dilation. Dorothy felt that this was the first act of betrayal by the medical staff. As soon as the internal exam is performed on a woman with ruptured membranes, her baby is at risk for developing an infection.

Dorothy was told she was three centimeters dilated and could not go home. She told me that she did not mind the pain of the contractions, and said her body really worked with them. After being in the hospital for some hours and dilating to five centimeters, the midwife wanted to start Pitocin to induce more dilation. Dorothy felt she was being pressured by doctors to speed up the labor because it had been a long time since her membranes had ruptured. When they began to discuss Pitocin, Dorothy's labor slowed down.

At this time Dorothy called me. She was crying as she told me she thought she was a failure because she had agreed to let the physician administer Pitocin. I asked her if she could tell herself she was not a failure. Could she surrender to the situation and not punish herself? She said she could, and that she felt slightly better.

In a postpartum visit, with her healthy four-month-old baby boy in her arms, Dorothy talked to me about the birth. She said she felt really "in control" while she labored drug-free. Her body surrendered to the contractions, which she did not experience as very painful. Once the Pitocin was started and she was being continuously monitored she felt "like I was in battle." Dorothy felt that the midwife had betrayed her trust by strongly suggesting that she take Pitocin and that she in turn had betrayed her baby. I asked her what she meant by her betrayal of her baby. She responded that since she had communicated with the midwives about her desire for a natural birth without the use of interventions such as Pitocin, she felt the midwife had betrayed her by agreeing with the physician to attempt the induction with the medication. Although the nurse encouraged her to have an epidural, Dorothy chose to decline any more medical intervention.

Continuing with her birth story, Dorothy related that after she had been pushing for a few hours she began to cry. The midwife asked her why she was crying and instructed her to continue pushing. Dorothy told me she felt very angry and that she believed that her anger gave her the energy to continue trying to push her baby out. This feeling scared her because it reminded her of a very old feeling of rage she remembered having as a child. She thought perhaps it was this memory of childhood anger that scared her and caused her to cry. She said the anger felt so very powerful. She cried while telling me about feeling so angry and betrayed.

Dorothy pushed for six hours before giving birth to her baby. I reminded her that she was allowed to push for six hours because she was under the care of a midwife. Without a supportive midwife present, most physicians would have performed a cesarean section after two or three hours of pushing.

After Peter was born, he was taken away from her for tests and observation. Several hours later, Dorothy went to find her baby so that she could spend time with him and nurse him.

Dorothy was upset that she did not have the birth she had wanted, free of medical intervention. She said, "I allowed Peter to go through a violent birth by taking the Pitocin." She, like many women, felt that she had failed because she had a Pitocin-induced labor.

I felt her birth was an act of strength and bravery and suggested that she try to forgive herself for not having the birth she had hoped for. I respected Dorothy for knowing exactly what she wanted for the birth, discussing it with her midwives, being strong, and allowing herself to experience her feelings. She had succeeded in birthing her baby after six arduous hours of pushing with no pain-relief medication. Dorothy said that she felt better after telling me her story. I encouraged her to voice her feelings with the midwives when she felt ready to do so.

Kelly's Story

Kelly was sixteen years old and pregnant with her first baby when she first came to me for childbirth preparation at the suggestion of her chiropractor. A well-informed and very bright teenager, she had been under the care of the chiropractor as her primary health care provider for many years.

Kelly and I planned a series of four private sessions. During the classes, I helped prepare Kelly and her boyfriend for labor and becoming parents. When I suggested labor support, she was very interested. They met with and arranged for a trainee who was studying to become a certified childbirth educator to assist them during labor. With the emotional support of her boyfriend and labor assistant, Kelly had a vaginal birth after a long hospital labor.

Six years later, Kelly came again to meet with me, pregnant with her second child. She had changed obstetricians. We talked about her life at this time and some of her experiences over the past six years. She told me about the strong, loving relationship she had with her mother.

I asked Kelly to tell me about her first birth experience. She had labored in the hospital for twenty-two hours, and had endured many internal exams and being watched by medical students. When she was offered an epidural, she declined, wanting a natural birth. Eventually, she had a forceps delivery after being told they "couldn't find the heartbeat." They took the baby away from her immediately after the birth. The baby was fine.

Kelly had kept all the educational material I had given her six years before and was rereading it. She knew that for this birth she did not want medical students in the room and wanted few internal examinations. We discussed her speaking to her new obstetrician about her choices for this birth. We reviewed the stages of labor and the transition to having a second baby. Kelly was concerned about her daughter's adjustment to the new baby and I suggested ways to help her prepare to become a big sister. Kelly had decided to hire the labor assistant who had supported her during the first labor.

Kelly spoke with her obstetrician about her desires for labor and delivery. When she told him she wanted to labor at home as long as possible, he cautioned that second labors are usually faster than first. Kelly responded that she "trusts her body" and would know when to leave for the hospital. Her obstetrician was pleased about her decision to have labor support.

Kelly was thrilled with the second birth, feeling more knowledgeable and empowered because of her first birth experience. She noted that the obstetrician was more respectful of her than the previous obstetrician. After the birth, Kelly sent me this note:

> Knowledge is the best gift someone can give and you gave us so much that we had the confidence to have this baby our way.

THE CARE PROVIDER

It is important to seek out a care provider, either a physician or a midwife, who values the pregnant woman's opinions and wishes regarding the birth experience. Interviewing the potential care provider is suggested for couples prior to making this critical decision. Most benefit from a referral from a trusted health professional or friend. Ideally, the care provider spends adequate time during prenatal visits addressing questions and concerns. Even in this era of managed care, some choice of health care provider and facility exists for most pregnant women. Especially now, women need to be encouraged to take responsibility for the choices available to them as health care consumers.

In the medical model the obstetrician is trained to be the authority figure who is responsible for the treatment of the patient. In contrast, midwives see themselves as teachers to help guide the pregnant woman and her family. A physician and a midwife perform the same physical screening procedures at a prenatal visit, but the midwife usually spends more time with the woman than the physician does. The midwife often asks the pregnant woman about how she is feeling emotionally as well as physically. In general, women who engage midwives for their prenatal care are encouraged to take greater responsibility for their pregnancies and births. They are actively given the opportunity to state their preferences for pain management, surgical intervention such as episiotomy, and other important considerations (Korte, 1997; Rothman, 1991).

Midwives offer the type of care that supports the pregnant woman in taking an active role in her childbirth experience. Midwife and author Penfield Chester writes, "The holistic model holds that birth is a normal, woman-centered process in which mind and body are one and that, in the vast majority of cases, nature is sufficient to create healthy pregnancy and birth. The midwife is seen as a nurturer" (Chester, 1997, p. 7). She describes the nurse-midwife and the independent or lay midwife as two different choices for midwifery care. The certified nurse-midwife offers an important option for women who desire to deliver their babies in the hospital or birth center. In most settings the nurse-midwife is an integral member of the obstetrics community. Chester writes, "The independent midwife reminds us of our allegiance to women, to homebirth, and to midwifery as an autonomous profession that honors and respects the wisdom of women's bodies and sets its own standards for their care" (1997, p. 278).

Studies have shown that women who are attended by nurse-midwives have a significantly lower chance of having a cesarean section than women who are attended by an obstetrician (Korte, 1997). In 1997, a study in Washington state found that women seen by certified nurse-midwives had a cesarean rate of 8.8 percent while women seen by obstetricians had a cesarean rate of 13.6 percent (Korte, 1997, p. 92). In other studies, all women had a lower chance of cesarean section with a nurse-midwife present, while the most dramatic reduction of cesarean was for VBAC women who were under the care of nurse-midwives (Korte, 1997). A 1998 study by the National Center for Health Statistics investigated one million normal vaginal deliveries, comparing birth outcomes in babies delivered by physicians and certified nurse-midwives. The data found that, when compared to births attended by physicians, those attended by certified nurse-midwives had significantly lower rates of infant death, neonatal mortality (an infant death that occurs in the first twenty-eight days of life), and low birthweight. In 1995, certified nurse-midwives delivered 6 percent of all births in the United States compared to 3 percent in 1989 (MacDorman and Singh, 1998). In Japan, Denmark, Sweden, and Holland, countries with low perinatal mortality rates, most births are attended by midwives.

THE WOMAN LISTENING
TO HER INNER WISDOM

As the woman prepares for the birth of her baby, she can become empowered by looking inward for guidance. She may have questions about issues that present themselves during pregnancy such as her changing identity at home and within the workplace. In addition to the support offered by the care provider and childbirth educator, a woman needs encouragement to trust her own instincts. She can access her inner strength and any spiritual connection that exists for her. This is often accomplished by quieting herself and listening for the answers within her. The following tools are helpful to the pregnant woman in listening to and trusting her own wisdom.

Meditation and Visualization

Meditation and visualization are valuable tools to calm fears experienced by many pregnant women and their partners. I incorporate these exercises into childbirth preparation, both group and individual, where I assist participants to access this form of relaxation. I lead participants in a meditation to help them relax and clear their minds of stress. I suggest that they close their eyes and take deep breaths, focusing on their inhalation and exhalation. I also ask them to focus on specific areas of the body, being aware of any tension and letting it go through the process of breathing. For women, I may proceed to a visualization of the baby growing healthy and strong inside of them. Another visualization involves guiding a client to imagine herself in a safe place where she can relax and enjoy the scene she has created. I encourage clients to use these meditations at home.

The meditation and visualization sessions differ between individual and group classes. An individual session utilizes an exercise specific to the needs of the client; for a woman who has had a cesarean section, I may lead her through a visualization of having a vaginal birth. In the class setting I address more general issues as described above. Christine, a client whose story appears in Chapters 8 and 9, benefited a great deal from our individual sessions, finding the visualizations calming and inspiring. She practiced meditation and visualization on her own during times of great fear and stress.

Karen's Story:
Making a Change During Pregnancy

Karen attended prenatal exercise classes that I was teaching. One night after class, she spoke to me about her anxiety regarding her decision to change from an obstetrics practice to a midwifery practice in another hospital. She chose to leave obstetricians who were affiliated with the hospital that employed her husband. For many reasons, she felt that being cared for by midwives would improve her childbirth experience. Though her husband supported her decision to change care providers, he was upset because he thought her choice might affect his job. Karen found making this decision quite stressful. She knew she had made the right choice for herself but feared it had left her husband in an uncomfortable position at work.

During her thirty-sixth week of pregnancy, the baby was in a breech position. She was concerned that if the baby's position did not change, an obstetrician would need to be present at the birth. For a breech presentation, most obstetricians perform a cesarean section.

I suggested that Karen practice relaxation exercises, quiet herself, and be assured that she had made the best choice for her pregnancy. I asked if she could let go of pleasing her husband and allow him to deal with his issues at work. She believed she could try to let go of his discomfort. I talked to her about letting herself feel safe and peaceful in the care of the midwives she had chosen. The baby moved into the correct position in the next few days and four weeks later she went on to give birth vaginally to a healthy baby.

In this case, Karen chose the type of care provider she needed. Although this decision caused her and her husband stress, the act of speaking about her ambivalence and anxiety helped her to relax and proceed with the birth of the baby.

Keeping a Journal

A helpful tool for a woman to utilize during pregnancy is keeping a journal. Writing is useful to sort through the many emotions that may emerge as well as a means to record the details of the process. If a woman is afraid or has other painful emotions, the act of journaling can be a way to release them. She may find the writing time helps her gain insight into the source of her anxiety. Although she may be resistant to spending the time writing in a journal, she may enjoy the quiet, contemplative time that it gives her. She may then want to discuss her concerns more openly, or find that they have decreased merely from the act of writing them down.

During the postpartum period, I encourage a client to write her birth story. If she is able to write the story soon after the birth, she tends to describe her emotions and the chronology of events. This exercise can be particularly useful after a traumatic birth or in a situation when the birth did not meet her expectations. Writing can enable her to begin to let go of her pain and disappointment, and approach mothering with a sense of wholeness.

Telling Her Story

I always suggest that a woman who has experienced a traumatic birth tell me her birth story. Many women comment that it is helpful to tell the story to an impartial listener. Dorothy, whose story is told earlier in this chapter, was feeling distraught about the use of medical intervention during the birth of her son. At a postpartum visit with me, she related her feelings about the birth experience. I encouraged her to speak with her midwife about it. I received a letter from Dorothy as I was writing this book. In it, she describes her experience of working through her anger by talking with her midwife:

I was very angry, after [Peter's] birth, about my experiences, after being induced. One of my midwives . . . said I needed to integrate the experience into my life. I couldn't even think about it, I'd get too angry. When Peter was about 26 months old, I went for my yearly check-up. The midwife who was with me through [Peter's] birth saw me and had lots of time or she made lots of time for me. We shared about that birth experience. It was wonderful. She shared what she went through. I shared my experience and feelings. Then she went on to tell about the changes in the midwife program at the hospital, that happened as a result of that birth (just little stuff); but, I walked away feeling like I was part of the solution instead of all of the problem. I have no anger today when I think about my birth experience. It is part of who my son is. I'm so grateful I was able to revisit and share my birth experience. It looks so wonderful when I don't have to see it through those angry glasses.

Once a woman has given birth, her story deserves to be told. Whether she shares her birth story with her childbirth educator, labor assistant, midwife, obstetrician, friend, or relative, the telling can be powerful and therapeutic for her.

THE PARTNER

The pregnant woman's partner provides support and strength by being involved in preparation for childbirth. Some partners accompany the woman to her prenatal visits. Attending childbirth classes together as a couple encourages communication with one another and with other couples. Couples who prepare for labor and birth together generally enjoy the sessions as a special time in their relationship.

During childbirth classes, one partner in the group may admit fears about the unknown experience of childbirth and how to help the woman when she is in pain. As another participant acknowledges the same fears, each begins to feel supported. The following are suggestions for partners to consider when trying to help the laboring woman. Reassuring words that she is doing well coping with the pain of labor, breathing, and even groaning with the laboring woman provides emotional connection. Gentle touch is an excellent form of physical support that a partner can provide during labor. Although the partner does not experience the pain, he or she will be of most comfort to the woman by being attentive, patient, and loving.

Partners also have needs for support while approaching this milestone in their own lives. In *Finding Our Fathers: How a Man's Life Is Shaped by His Relationship with His Father,* psychologist Samuel Osherson (1986) writes of his own journey during his wife's pregnancy. In talking about the husband's role, he states, "Yet the fact that only the woman experiences the unique reality of being physically pregnant need not detract from or negate the fact that the husband needs information, reassurance, and support as he explores this mysterious part of life and constructs for himself the new role of Father, a major life transition" (p. 173).

A man experiences many changes as he prepares to be a father. For many men socialized to "be tough," it can be difficult to explore their own needs. A man may be worried about the health of his wife and the developing baby. Some men decide to attend to their own health in ways they have not done prior to the pregnancy to ensure they will be able to provide physically, financially, and emotionally for the new family. A common theme for the father-to-be is that only the pregnant woman, not himself, is in need of support.

Men can experience great opportunities for their own growth and healing during the pregnancy and postpartum period. Jack Heinowitz, author of *Pregnant Fathers: Entering Parenthood Together* (1995), reflects, "Ultimately, fathers *themselves* must take responsibility for healing their wounds and creating a healthy, nonviolent world. . . . For a man to willingly wrap himself in the cloak of fatherhood, he must first go inward and begin to love himself" (p. 65).

LABOR SUPPORT FROM ANOTHER WOMAN

Couples may hire a professional labor assistant, a doula, to give them added emotional and physical support during labor. According to a number of studies, constant support by another woman during labor, whether professional or not, decreases the risk of cesarean section, the use of pain medication, and of anesthesia. The assisted women also had more interest in their newborns than those without this support (Klaus, Kennell, and Klaus, 1993, p. 34).

A study of 412 healthy women in labor in a U.S. hospital showed that providing support during labor resulted in positive outcomes for mothers and babies (Kennell et al., 1991). Participants of the study were assigned to either a support person or an unobtrusive observer. An additional 204 women were assigned to a control group with no changes from standard medical practice. The study found that continuous labor support significantly decreased the rate of cesarean section deliveries (supported group, 8 percent; observed group, 13 percent; and control group, 18 percent). Forceps deliveries were lowered. Epidural anesthesia for spontaneous vaginal deliveries was also reduced in the supported women (supported group, 7.8 percent; observed group, 22.6 percent; and control group, 55.3 percent). Pitocin use, duration of labor, prolonged infant hospitalization, and maternal fever were all decreased in the supported group.

Childbirth is a time when women have a special place in each other's lives. I recommend that all women enlist the support of another woman during labor and delivery. The companion could be a midwife, a labor assistant, or a caring friend or relative of the laboring woman. For those interested in hiring a labor assistant, the most important factor is that the pregnant woman and her partner feel comfortable with and nurtured by this woman.

The labor assistant provides support and suggestions to encourage the woman during the course of labor. She can be especially helpful during a period in which the labor has slowed down or stopped. Suggestions include the woman changing position, walking, taking nourishment, showering, resting, sleeping, or talking. Talking about her feelings is extremely important and helpful. The woman may need to talk about her fears of the pain of contractions. She may be anxious about birthing the baby and becoming a mother. Reassurance about her feelings can allow the laboring woman to relax and proceed with the birthing process. While working with Sara (her story is told in Chapter 8), I spoke with her for a long time as she rested in a bathtub when her labor had slowed down considerably. She expressed some feelings about the loss of her mother at an early age. Later that day, her labor intensified and she was able to have a vaginal birth.

Women often share with me their intense fear of the birth process. Though the pain of contractions may be frightening, they need to be encouraged that it is this pain that brings about the birth of the baby. During labor, a woman must be encouraged to surrender to the pain. Emotional encouragement from the labor assistant empowers a woman during labor. Positive messages from the birth attendants that her labor is progressing as it should and that she is doing a great job are helpful in maintaining the desired progress of labor.

Dina's Story

> For me it's very natural to have a special feeling for you. You helped me give birth, like a sister.

After having a traumatic cesarean section for her first birth, Dina researched having a vaginal birth (VBAC). She and her husband read Nancy Wainer Cohen's book, *Silent Knife* (Cohen and Estner, 1983) while she was pregnant with the second baby. They contacted the author, who referred them to me for labor support. When I first met with Dina, it was apparent that both she and her husband were well-informed about VBAC. She had selected an obstetrician who delivered in a hospital a good distance from her home because of his progressive attitude toward VBAC and his respect for and support of his patients.

Dina and her husband are strictly observant Jews. In the Jewish faith, Friday sundown to Saturday sundown is the Sabbath, Shabbat, a time of rest. For Dina and her husband, the observance of Shabbat includes avoiding work, the use of electricity, and the use of the telephone. Driving in a car is forbidden, as is spending money. Because of their concerns about the labor beginning during this holy day, Dina's husband had checked with a trusted rabbi about using the telephone should she go into labor on Shabbat. He replied that it would be acceptable to use the telephone during Shabbat to call me for labor support.

Dina's labor began on a Saturday morning. Though she had been given permission to contact me on Shabbat, she did not feel that the birth was imminent, and chose to labor on her own all that day. She did not call me until that evening after sundown. Dina exhibited a profound strength in her ability to labor unsupported because of the importance of her religious values.

I drove with Dina and her husband to the hospital and remained there with her for many hours during the long labor. I supported her as she gave birth by VBAC to a healthy baby boy.

Dina formed a strong connection to me because I helped her have her baby without major abdominal surgery. Dina's own words describe the power of the support she received:

> Sitting in the car with my husband driving us to the hospital, having you in the car, I thought, I am not alone . . . to have someone near me to help me, to have you was so much help for both of us . . . especially me. It was so much help for me . . .
>
> To have you there in the hospital was very, very helpful because I was in so much pain . . . to know I was not alone. It was absolutely crucial to have you . . . you were holding my hand, telling me I was doing fine . . . seeing you made me believe I can do it . . . it is very important to ask G-d for help but to feel the help, to have people to help. . . . Listening to your words was very calming . . . it was frightening for me, having you was crucial . . . to my knowing I could do it. . . . Seeing the progress in me was very important, I didn't know because I was in so much pain. So also after I gave birth to my children, I felt an especially close feeling to you, reassured by your word and deed, an intense feeling after I gave birth . . . closeness to you. Afterwards, to have a healthy baby . . . I felt very close to you. A normal birth, a healthy baby . . . Giving birth naturally is so different from having a cesarean section. Actually, having a natural birth makes you a woman, then being able to nurse the baby. I was so sick after the cesarean and I was in terrible pain. Natural birth makes a woman . . . it's very personal . . . I want you to know I always remember you . . . I think of you . . . You helped me give birth.

After the birth, Dina came to consider me an important source of support, "like a sister" to her. I subsequently provided labor support for her next vaginal birth. Dina went on to have a family of five healthy children, all but the first one vaginal births.

When I attend a birth, I encourage the laboring woman to stay in the present time, feeling one contraction at a time. I affirm that she is working hard and coping with the painful sensations. While giving her physical and emotional support, she knows that I will remain with her as long as she needs me. I encourage her to change positions, to take a shower, to use the different tools available to her to get through this very long, hard process of labor and giving birth. We talk if she wants to talk, and are quiet if that is more appropriate.

Maura's Story

After having her first child by cesarean section, Maura and her husband attended my VBAC classes. She had a homebirth VBAC and was thrilled with her experience. A few years later, I was asked by Maura to attend the homebirth of her next child.

Maura, a petite, athletic woman, was over a week past her due date when her labor began. She called me and I arrived at her home at about 11:30 p.m. She was in active labor. After a few contractions, I asked if she had called her midwife. Maura had not yet called and asked me to do so. I spoke to the midwife, describing the labor, and she stated that she was on her way.

Whenever Maura began to feel a contraction, she walked across the room and leaned against her piano, standing there for the entire contraction. It was a powerful image to witness because she walked during contractions as if she had a destination. After the contraction, she rested for a minute. As soon as another contraction began, she walked and leaned again. I kept telling her that she was doing extremely well. Maura's husband was asleep, as were her children. She seemed quite content as she surrendered to the pain and concentrated inward for her strength.

The midwives and apprentice arrived. They evaluated Maura's progress by observing her. No mention was ever made of performing an internal exam. I was struck by the respect and calm afforded to Maura by the midwives. Labor was progressing quickly when Maura asked if she could take a bath. The midwife replied that she could and Maura requested that I accompany her and pour water over her abdomen while she was in the tub. After being in the tub for just a few minutes, Maura began to grunt. The midwife who was standing in the doorway calmly said, "Let's get you out of the tub, this baby is going to be coming soon."

The midwife had set up her sterile area in the living room, Maura's husband had been awakened, and the other midwife had arrived. We helped Maura walk into the living room and she began to push. After a few pushes, her baby was born at 2:30 a.m. Her husband woke the other children to come in and meet their new sister. It was a peaceful and beautiful birth.

Cindy's Births

I had the privilege of helping my sister Cindy twice as she labored and gave birth to her daughters. During these two special births, I supported my sister and her husband as Cindy labored and gave birth to their children, Allison and Jennifer. My mother, father, and other sister were present for the birth of Jennifer, the younger daughter. My father shared that this was an amazing event for him since, like other men of his generation, he was not allowed to participate in the births of his own daughters. In a letter to me he wrote:

> I pay you a debt of gratitude for receiving the benefits of your pursuits and writing in this field which for me, culminated in my being present at the birth of your sister Cindy's second child, my granddaughter Jennifer. This was a unique experience in my life, one of the greatest moments that I will never forget. Finally, this gave me the privilege of being present at and seeing what I can only describe as the "miracle of birth," a God given moment.

As a woman gives birth, the pushing out of her baby is a wondrous moment in which time stands still. Some births are long and seemingly endless, and others are quick, just as a woman's healing may take years or may occur in a shorter span of time. Birth is the power of the woman letting go, surrendering to the vast array of sensations and feelings that exist. As one of the assistants in this momentous event, seeing the birth of a baby take place before my eyes is a joy that is indescribable.

PART IV:
BIRTH AS A HEALING EXPERIENCE

Chapter 6

Vaginal Birth
After Cesarean (VBAC)

*We believe that birth is a natural process that can take place
naturally. We believe that every pregnant woman can give birth if
she so desires and has the proper information and support. Every
woman can find the strength from within to deliver her baby as
she integrates feelings of trust and confidence in her body, ac-
cepts her particular labor, and appreciates the process of birth.*

Nancy Wainer Cohen and Lois J. Estner
*Silent Knife: Cesarean Prevention
and Vaginal Birth After Cesarean,*
1983, p. 3.

One of my goals as a childbirth educator and counselor is to foster
an awareness of the emotional issues present during pregnancy, childbirth, and the postpartum period. In my private practice, I provide an
opportunity for a woman to feel her emotions. She has the time to
mourn her losses. I am concerned that unprocessed grief, fear, or anger
may emerge as symptoms of depression, anxiety, or physical ailments
which may have negative effects on a woman's pregnancy or mothering experience. I listen to and accept a woman's story of emotional
pain. It is in this compassionate and empathic witnessing that I help a
woman to proceed in her life.

PREPARATION FOR VBAC

A woman who has given birth by cesarean section and wishes to
have a vaginal birth benefits enormously by preparing for the up-

63

coming birth. I counsel women who have a range of feelings about their experiences of giving birth by cesarean section. In assisting them to prepare for a vaginal birth after cesarean (VBAC), I help them deal with the sometimes painful emotional scars remaining from the surgical birth. I believe that discussing the previous birth, as well as preparing for the next birth, is a process worth pursuing regardless of the type of delivery a woman goes on to have. I acknowledge that it takes courage to discuss the past birth experience and prepare for a VBAC. Support and education are very important and increase her chance of having a vaginal birth.

A woman who chooses individual VBAC preparation sessions is able to speak privately about the experience of her cesarean section and be supported for any issues that are still present for her. Many women think that only another woman who has had a cesarean section and VBAC can truly empathize with their experience. They feel that this shared experience is more real and believable than the thoughtful words given by family, friends, or health care professionals. Miriam Greenspan, therapist and author, writes in *A New Approach to Women and Therapy* (1983), "It is a matter of sharing, where appropriate, the understanding of their problems that comes from my own experience; of expressing empathy where their own pain touches on mine. . . . Connecting with clients in these and other ways often helps them to see themselves in a new way" (p. 244).

It is common for women who have had cesarean births to say they have no feelings about the birth except relief that the baby is healthy. Women admit that they feel selfish if they complain about the birth experience, instead of just feeling grateful that the baby is fine. I explain that it is not selfish to have their own feelings about their birth experiences. They are entitled to feel disappointment at the same time that they feel gratitude and joy.

Pregnancy can trigger intense feelings of anxiety, anger, or guilt that have not been sufficiently resolved following the previous cesarean. Because women do not usually deal with their feelings shortly after a cesarean section, I find that when preparing for a VBAC, they are often ready for and in need of grieving before the next birth. Processing the emotional aspects of their previous birth experiences can be an important part of their preparation for the subsequent pregnancy, labor, and postpartum period.

Understandably, women pursuing a VBAC often have a lot of resistance to VBAC preparation for fear they will "fail again." I assure a client that she did not fail; rather, she did her best under the circumstances. She may have been told that she needed a cesarean because her pelvis was too small, the labor got "stuck," or the baby was too large. She may have trouble believing that her body is capable of giving birth naturally because she has not yet experienced it. Some women state that they are disappointed in themselves because they could not cope with the pain of labor. A woman may be urged to "just listen to the doctor" by close family and friends, which leaves her feeling alone with her decision to attempt a VBAC.

Many women striving for a vaginal birth after cesarean feel ambivalent about committing to and obtaining support for it. They may come for a session at the very end of the pregnancy when there is insufficient time for me to educate them. When a client meets with me in the final weeks of her pregnancy, she may not be able to fully process her fear and anxiety about a VBAC, and her ambivalence may impair her ability to feel secure in her decisions about the upcoming birth.

A woman preparing to have a VBAC came to me for one session in the thirty-seventh week of her pregnancy. With her first pregnancy, which resulted in a cesarean section, she had labored at home for a time before going to the hospital. At the hospital, having dilated to four centimeters, she was given Pitocin by her doctor because, according to him, she was not dilating quickly enough. She then received an epidural for pain and proceeded to fully dilate. After pushing for thirty minutes, there was a question of fetal distress and a cesarean section was performed. When speaking to me, she related that she was upset about receiving the Pitocin and the epidural. She was sad that she had not been able to see her son for a long time after the birth.

She desired a vaginal birth so she could avoid the recovery of a cesarean section, and be better able to care for her newborn and her two-year-old. I told her that she could enlist the support she needed at this birth and make choices to help her cope with the pain. I encouraged her to have the strength to have a vaginal birth. She referred to herself as "a wimp, like my mother." I did not agree with this characterization of herself. She had fully dilated with the use of Pitocin, which intensified the labor. She had tried pushing her baby out but the physician decided she needed a cesarean.

I called to wish her well a few days prior to her due date. A woman identifying herself as the client's mother answered the telephone. She told me that her daughter had just had the baby the previous day by cesarean section. The mother stated that her daughter had "chickened out" in the last few days and requested a cesarean. The messages about pregnancy and childbirth that a pregnant woman receives from those close to her, her care providers, and from the surrounding culture have a powerful effect on her. Without adequate and timely support, the difficult choice of trying for a VBAC may not be possible.

Though the end of the pregnancy is not a time to begin the complex emotional work that can be involved in having a VBAC, it is a time when a woman can receive valuable support. I encourage clients to listen to their own needs, rest if necessary, and enjoy the time in any way that brings them comfort. Completing projects at work, though possibly stressful, may also provide relief as they approach the next phase of life. The weeks prior to delivery are an important time to spend with the partner and other children before the joyous arrival of an infant with its demands on the mother's time and energy.

Significant healing can take place between two women. During individual VBAC preparation, I generally suggest that my client and I begin with one or two sessions to become familiar with each other. If she desires to prepare for a VBAC without her partner, we continue to meet that way. A woman makes an individual choice to meet with me alone or with her partner. For each woman it is different. For some clients, VBAC preparation consists of individual support and guidance. For others, it is a time for the couple to spend time learning together.

CLIENTS' STORIES

After the initial history, I ask my client to tell me her experience of having a cesarean section. When I am working with the couple, I request that both partners describe their experiences of the cesarean birth. Not only does the telling of the story provide me with important information, it also allows time for both of them to speak about their experiences. Couples do not have the opportunity to tell their stories of disappointment, loss, and sadness often enough.

While telling me the story of her cesarean section, a woman may begin to remember and feel a wide range of emotions, including anger, shame, and grief. Many women sob when they recount their experiences. After the woman is finished, I assure her, if she seems embarrassed by her emotions, that crying is part of the healing process. For those who blame themselves for the cesarean, I encourage them to forgive themselves and let go of that which was beyond their control at the time.

The partner's story is also very important in order for the couple to work together to plan for the next birth. At times, the partner will share experiences of sadness or anger. After hearing the story, I speak about the importance and value of allowing these emotions to emerge as they approach and plan for the next birth. If a partner has specific concerns, fears, or anxieties about the upcoming birth, it is very helpful to discuss these issues. In another session I begin to talk to the couple about choices for the next birth. Making choices empowers them to avoid another cesarean section unless it is absolutely necessary. We discuss their needs and expectations for the forthcoming birth.

I am conscious of the importance of adults, especially women, being listened to in these busy times in which we live. Greenspan (1983) writes, "Traditionally, women have not been listened to very well. Our stories have not been heard or validated from our own point of view" (p. 240). Of the women I have helped prepare for a VBAC, all have said that their ability to speak and not be judged about their cesarean experience was very helpful.

In addition to discussing the previous birth, the suggestions for honoring the experience of childbirth presented in Chapter 5 are especially useful in preparing for a VBAC. Some couples are very interested in hiring labor support and others express resistance to this idea. I encourage clients to enlist helpful and kind support people so they are able to complete the difficult act of labor. A suggestion that I make for the woman who is experiencing a healthy pregnancy is to plan to stay home where she is free to labor and move around comfortably in her own surroundings during early labor. She can arrive at the hospital when she has a limited amount of time left to labor. I emphasize that there is no definite time for a woman to enter the hospital. Only she will know if she wants to stay home or finds she is ready to go to the hospital. Although I hope that a woman will not arrive at the hospital too early in the labor, it is important that she knows that it is her choice when to leave her home.

At the end of our sessions preparing for the upcoming birth, I emphasize the importance of having spent time and energy processing and healing from a previous birth experience. Together we have planned for a vaginal birth, but in the event a woman has another cesarean, I encourage her to credit herself for the time and effort she spent in preparing for the birth.

Sheila's Story: Repeat Cesarean After Attempted VBAC—Satisfaction with the Birth Experience

Sheila and her husband Jon came to prepare for a VBAC during her second pregnancy, at the suggestion of her prenatal exercise instructor. Sheila had given birth to her first baby by cesarean section four years earlier. The baby was born in a large teaching hospital and weighed over nine pounds. She did not see her baby for several hours after the cesarean and did not nurse him for twenty-four hours. She always wondered if he was a poorly nursing baby because of this delay in nursing. For the first birth, she had chosen to be under the care of a high-risk obstetrics practice because of her history of respiratory problems.

At the time she was preparing for her VBAC, Sheila believed she did not need to be at a high-risk practice because of her medical condition. She changed care providers and planned to give birth to this baby vaginally, with a woman physician, at another hospital.

I spoke to Sheila and Jon about the issues present during the first birth. She had experienced a cesarean section, and was not able to see her baby or nurse him for many hours after he was born. During her first session, she told me that her mother had died when she was young. I encouraged her to come for more sessions to discuss this very important loss in her life. Sheila responded that she did not want to talk about this issue again. At her second and final visit, she wanted to "just prepare for the birth." We discussed the possible progress of a VBAC labor and techniques to cope with painful contractions.

Sheila and Jon hired a labor assistant to be with them for the labor and birth. Although Sheila dilated fully during this labor, she did have another cesarean section. For Sheila, even though the second labor was much more intense and painful than the first, she felt much better about the birth experience and about herself after giving birth. She was pleased that she did the best she possibly could in laboring a long time, spending time in the shower, and having a labor support person present. Jon was also satisfied with the birth, and content that Sheila dilated fully and labored as long as she was able to before having the cesarean section. Even though Sheila did not have a vaginal birth, she felt much more empowered and content after her second cesarean than she had after her first.

Marcia's Story: VBAC

During her second pregnancy, Marcia came to meet with me individually to gain support for a VBAC. She had given birth to Jessica four and a half years before by cesarean section.

Marcia, a health care professional, felt she knew more about the risks and complications of pregnancy than the average woman. She told me that during her first pregnancy and labor, she had been very nervous about the pain of labor. Toward the end of her first pregnancy, Marcia had developed preeclampsia.* She was placed on bed rest for a while. In her thirty-sixth week of pregnancy, labor was induced for a short time and then she had a cesarean section. Jessica weighed four pounds at birth.

When Marcia told me the cesarean story, she expressed a lot of sorrow that she did not see or hold her baby at birth. She reported that the doctors were "cold, impersonal" and that she felt abandoned by her midwife. During the six-week postpartum visit, Marcia told her midwife that she was disappointed about her birth experience and they "had a good talk." She was upset telling me the story, more than four years later.

During her second pregnancy, as she began preparing for a VBAC, Marcia stated that she was not as nervous about pain as she had been during the first pregnancy. She had read informative childbirth books that she found helpful. She had hired labor support before coming to meet with me. She expected the labor to progress quickly. I cautioned her that VBAC labors often proceed slowly, warning her to be careful about her expectations. We reviewed labor signs. She was reassured to

---

*Preeclampsia, often called toxemia, is an illness during pregnancy in which a woman has high blood pressure, edema, protein in the urine, and often excessive weight gain. It affects between 5 and 10 percent of pregnant women and is more common during first pregnancies.

learn that I had had a VBAC and had endured a long transition stage. I urged her to be gentle with herself, and to tell herself that she could do it, she could have a VBAC. And she did.

The following are excerpts from Marcia's writing after her VBAC experience:

> My pregnancy was a healthy one and uneventful. I was nervous about labor pains and worried about the unknown throughout pregnancy and was therefore nervous about labor and delivery . . .
>
> I was so glad that Cheryl, a doula I hired for support, agreed to come to my house instead of meeting me at the birthing center. How would I have known when I was in active labor? How would I know how challenging labor would become? My family and I would have been nervous without Cheryl at our home and I probably would have gone to the birthing center prematurely. It's possible I may not have progressed so smoothly without this support . . .
>
> I felt very reassured by Cheryl's presence as if she knew what I was going through and knew what would come next. I am thrilled that I was able to continue to breathe, meditate and stay focused and relaxed with each subsequent contraction all the way to and at the birthing center.
>
> Driving to the birthing center: When I stepped out of her car I was greeted by a lovely, sincere, happy and centered face and I knew it was Claudia (the doula apprenticing with Cheryl). We had spoken two or three times previously and I agreed to have her participate at my birth. I immediately hugged her and I knew we were both happy to be with one another.
>
> I was greeted by my midwife Janet. . . . I was thrilled with my progression.
>
> Pushing: Cheryl was at my side near my face talking to me throughout the pushing and in between the contractions. She would tell me I was doing great, would remind me to relax and breathe in between, and to take a cleansing breath when I felt the contraction just beginning. . . . Eventually Janet suggested the birthing stool, which I was happy about, because I would be able to work with gravity and do something a little out of the ordinary.

I felt more in tune with mother earth being on the ground. Leaning back on Claudia . . . was supportive for it was a bit tiring holding myself up.

Finally out came Elissa. . . . Immediately after the birth, while still sitting on the stool . . . I held the crying, wet, pink-faced infant in my arms and had a nice long opportunity to hold her against my wet, warm, naked body . . . I stared at the baby savoring every moment. This had been my dream come true of a natural experience. She was normal, had all her body parts, and was crying loudly and continuously.

Thanks to my family, the doulas, the midwife, and my desire to have a normal, vaginal delivery, I was able to accomplish what millions of other women have also. It took courage, patience and trust in myself, trust in my support people, and trust in the universe.

The following story is another example of the value of woman-to-woman support, especially during a VBAC labor.

Rosa's Story: Value of Woman-to-Woman Support, VBAC

While in training to become a certified childbirth educator, I was required to attend and observe eight births. Rosa, a participant in my supervisor's childbirth preparation classes, was the first woman I assisted. During her ninth month, I met with her to discuss my support of her during her labor and birth. Rosa hoped and planned for a VBAC. During her cesarean section she had been very frightened because she felt that she had been all alone. As we talked, she told me how committed she was to avoiding another cesarean.

Ten days past her due date, Rosa's partner called me at 8:00 p.m. and told me that she had been in labor for one and a half hours and that she needed me. I later discovered that she had actually been in labor all day and had chosen to continue working at her place of business. When I arrived at her home at 8:35 p.m., her contractions were coming every minute and a half and lasting one minute. I, a friend who was also in training to be a childbirth educator, Rosa, and the twenty-year-old daughter of her partner drove to the hospital together in my car. Rosa's water broke in the car on the way to the hospital. Because her labor was so advanced, we went directly to the hospital emergency room on the advice of my supervisor. Rosa, a Latina woman, was speaking Spanish, her native language, during the intensity of her labor.

At 9:45 p.m. Rosa was fully dilated. The four of us in the emergency room, two Caucasian and two Latina women, were not communicating with each other verbally, yet were bonded together in the excitement of labor. No emotional support was given by the hospital attendants. Rosa looked to the nurse for help in the correct way to push. The nurse gave her no assistance or encouragement. I told Rosa to look at me, and I pushed with her.

The baby was crowning and ready to be born. Without explaining why, the resident took out surgical shears and performed an episiotomy. Rosa seemed more uncomfortable after the episiotomy than she was with the labor. Her daughter, Maria, was born at 10:30 p.m. in the emergency room. Rosa cried in pain as the resident sutured her and the placenta was delivered. She seemed dazed right after the birth.

Ten days later I paid Rosa a postpartum visit. She was thrilled with the birth and very proud of herself. Rosa stated that she had worked the entire day while experiencing contractions; it was only after coming home at 6:00 p.m. that she realized how close together the contractions were. Rosa commented that the doctors at the clinic where she received her prenatal care had informed her that she had a small pelvis and would not be able to have a VBAC. She had known in her heart that she wanted to try for a vaginal birth despite this information. Rosa was so pleased to have had the baby her way, without abdominal surgery.

Group VBAC Preparation

Group VBAC preparation classes help participants to prepare for the next birth by sharing similar experiences. My groups, three to five couples, meet for two-hour sessions every week for six weeks. Each group is distinct because every member has individual needs and expectations. Some individuals want to be instructed about ways to avoid another cesarean while others do not want to question the physician's authority. Some participants have a desire to talk about their cesarean experiences in the group setting while others do not.

People who choose to be part of a VBAC group tend to respect each other and try not to influence one another. They share their own issues and appreciate being listened to by their peers. If a member is hesitant to speak, I do not pressure her or him to do so. Many times a quiet member will share more openly in the third meeting than in the first two meetings, needing time to develop a sense of safety before speaking her or his feelings.

At one of the early sessions, I request that members tell their cesarean stories if they feel comfortable doing so. Women and men have shared very painful memories of their cesarean births with the group. Some members cry as they speak. Some participants speak about being angry that they or their partner had a cesarean that possibly could have been avoided. I note that they are entitled to experience all their emotions about the birth. The other group members listen attentively. Participants often remark that the act of telling their stories helped them accept their birth experiences as they occurred.

In some groups, questions are raised by members about the experience they have just heard and group discussion begins. We then progress to education about labor, electronic fetal monitoring, and other medical interventions. I use the guidelines I have discussed in Chapter 5 to educate VBAC couples. We end several classes of the series with meditation and visualization exercises. During a meditation session the participants close their eyes as I lead them through a scene of total relaxation. One of the visualization exercises is of the woman giving birth with the partner as a member of the support team.

I find VBAC groups to be very rewarding for me and empowering for the members. At the conclusion of the series, I reaffirm to the members that the process of meeting for a number of weeks, becoming educated, and speaking about their cesareans is important for their readiness for the upcoming birth. At the final session, we discuss the possibility that, even with all the preparation, a vaginal birth cannot be guaranteed. I encourage couples to speak about accepting themselves even if another cesarean is necessary and suggest they spend time with one another outside the class to talk about this topic.

The following story of Janet, a VBAC woman, is one of triumph and courage.

Janet's Story: Homebirth VBAC

During a prenatal exercise program that I led, I met Janet. When I scheduled a VBAC series, she and her husband enrolled. Janet's first baby had been born by cesarean section two years earlier for a breech presentation.

Janet wrote about her first pregnancy:

> In the eighth month of my first pregnancy I found out that our baby was breech. She stayed that way into my ninth month, so our doctor strongly advised me to have a C-section without labor. He said that at his hospital they had lost a breech baby that week because the mother had wanted to deliver her baby naturally; had she agreed to a C-section, he said, her baby would have lived. Scared stiff, I never thought of doing anything else.

Janet continued about her cesarean experience:

> I never had a labor pain. The experience was awful. The anesthetic didn't work. I was in excruciating pain, I couldn't move, and I was terrified. Once our daughter was pulled out, the anesthetist gave me Demerol and I went out of it. Someone brought Katie over to me, but I couldn't hold her; my arms were stretched out and strapped down with an IV and a cuff to gauge my blood pressure. I was scared and distraught.

Nearly two years later, Janet reported that, when she found out she was pregnant again, the fear from that first delivery returned. Her obstetrician told her she was "high risk" and that she would have to be placed on a fetal heart monitor and watched closely as soon as she went into labor. Janet was surprised and troubled because she had never even had a labor pain in the last pregnancy. In Janet's mind, she was a healthy and physically fit pregnant woman. She wondered why, if this baby was in the right position and her pregnancy was normal, she would be high risk.

Janet told me she wanted to have a natural birth, but didn't think to question the doctors until speaking with me. Janet and her husband George took the VBAC classes, began reading informative childbirth books, and began to advocate for their upcoming birth. They decided to interview new obstetricians and ultimately changed physicians but remained with the same hospital because of the limits of their insurance coverage. The new obstetrician encouraged them to have a VBAC, yet outlined procedures that they felt were a setup for another cesarean. Janet would be placed on constant fetal monitoring once admitted to the hospital in labor. She would have a heparin lock inserted in her arm (for an IV needle if needed on short notice) in the event she needed medication or surgery. She had voiced her desire to be able to walk around freely during her labor, with which the obstetrician had agreed. She realized that this would be impossible if she were immobilized by the external fetal monitor.

After expressing their concerns to their doctor about the medical interventions, he replied that he was obligated to follow hospital policy. Janet and George realized then that they would not be able to have their baby their way with this doctor and decided to seek out a new care provider. George tried but was unable to change insurance companies. They approached an obstetrician well-known for his support of midwives and natural childbirth, who agreed to take them into his practice during Janet's ninth month of pregnancy. Janet could give birth with the nurse-midwives of the practice. Janet and George were concerned about the financial cost, especially if complications developed.

Janet and George eventually decided to have their baby at home with the lay midwife they had already hired to provide labor support. They trusted and respected this midwife and her assistant and they believed in the safety and self-fulfillment of having their baby at home. They met with their midwife to discuss how to prepare their home, problems that could arise during labor, techniques to deal with minor issues, and procedures for an emergency.

This is an excerpt from Janet's account of her second birth experience:

> At home I was at peace, allowing my body to give birth the way it wanted to. In the thirty-five hours of my labor, I was never frightened or worried about my previous C-section causing problems. Not even in the last intense hour, when the contractions were coming back to back, was I worried. Peggy and her partner [the midwives] were wonderful, calm, competent, and supportive.
>
> At 7:30 that Friday night, I was having a cup of tea in bed and holding our daughter Suzanne who had been born at the side of my bed a half hour earlier. I was happier than I had ever been. I have never wanted anything more than I wanted to

have the *right* to have Suzanne normally. I could have accepted a C-section if I had thought for one moment that it was best for her. But I wanted the right to choose for myself. I had fought for that right and won.

I remember lying on my back, Suzanne on my tummy, her cord still uncut, moments after she had been born. I kept repeating, "I did it. I did it."

Peggy looked at me and replied, "Yes, Janet. *You* did it."

The following is George's account of this experience.

George's Story

If it were to be in chronological order, I'd start with driving to the hospital with Janet two and a half years earlier for the birth of our first child, knowing ahead of time that we would have a new baby delivered at 8:30 in the morning, *if* the doctors and surgeons were running on schedule. It was no different than driving to an airport to pick up a passenger at a precise arrival time, *if* the plane was running on schedule. That's how elective surgery works, good, bad, or indifferent.

The predictability didn't of itself make it such a bad thing, I suppose. But there was to be a delivery whether Janet went into labor or not, and as I stood by the operating table on the other side of a white sheet hearing her moan and cry in pain because, as I later learned, the anesthetic hadn't worked before the surgeon started cutting, I had little experience or reason to know or to sense just how unnecessary and traumatic this type of delivery was. Certainly I had no time to think about it, because suddenly a baby was handed over the white cloth, put into an incubator on wheels, and I was led out of the room behind it and the nurse and away from my wife, who went back into surgery not to be seen for several hours. What had happened bothered me, but in the confusion of it all, including the excitement of having a new baby, it came and largely went. Only over time did I realize how much it had affected Janet.

Two years later, we met you [Lois]. Janet was pregnant and determined never to endure or accept what had happened during her first pregnancy. I was along for the ride. What a ride.

That's the back-story. Now shift forward eight months from when we met you [Lois]. On a warm, sunny day, I'm looking out the window . . . looking up, then down to Janet at the edge of the bed, then up again . . . every ten seconds. Downstairs in the kitchen, the steam is rising from the pot where the utensils have been sterilizing for a half hour at least in boiling water because I can't get downstairs to turn the stove off. Looking down I can see the top of the baby's head, I think, beginning to emerge, but looking up, I can't see the midwife in the driveway yet, so I'm nervous, but confident and so is Janet.

We're not in a hospital. We chose to be at home, or at least to stay at home unless unforeseen circumstances and the midwives' judgment dictate that we do otherwise. But that's secondary to this story, as are the midwives who are on the way like the cavalry and would arrive just in time. Whether in the hospital or at home, with nurses or midwives, what is most important is that Janet, moaning and gasping at the edge of the bed, is getting the chance she was denied when our first baby was born without a labor pain. Now she is having a trial of labor . . . something that her doctor at the HMO said was too risky, not because she wasn't healthy or had had a troubled pregnancy before, but because she had had a C-section that first time and thus was at risk this second time, and therefore, should not be allowed to undergo a trial of labor.

To have a chance, a chance denied once before, to try, to try together—though I am definitely the lesser—more coach and fan than player—is something that we believe will make this baby and her mother healthier and happier, and will draw us closer together. For Janet, especially, but for me too this has turned into an act of affirming what we believe in and asserting our principles and ourselves.

The pain, Janet says, is excruciating . . . it is also transforming. The midwives arrive minutes beforehand, calm and competent. With Janet at the side of the bed, I try to coach and encourage, watching in awe. There is no white curtain between us. Knowing much more than I did the first time, I know the difference in the sounds of pain I hear now and heard then. Instead of the baby being taken, the baby is being given by her body. Whether Janet succeeds or not in having this baby naturally and at home, without surgery or complications—and we are both prepared without hesitation to go to the hospital and she to undergo surgery if the midwives recommend or Janet decides [it is] best—she has tried on her own terms and that will be one of the single greatest steps of personal growth she has ever taken.

I watch in disbelief as Janet pushes out one last time and quietly there emerges our new daughter looking about with wide open eyes, so silent I fear she is not breathing. The midwives give the baby to Janet to hold, something she couldn't do and didn't care to do when our first baby was born and she was in excruciating pain. The look on Janet's face speaks of two dreams achieved. While the midwives clean up, Janet and I and our new daughter, Suzanne, lie in our bed together. Soon one of the midwives will bring tea, some cheese and crackers, and for me, a bottle of beer. Then they will perform thorough tests and measurements on Suzanne, more thorough by the way than anything the doctor at the HMO did the next day when we were told to bring the baby. But that was another day.

Lying in bed with Janet and our new baby that day, I looked out the window for the first time since the midwives arrived and saw that indeed it was a warm, sunny day. Inside our bedroom, beside us, and inside the two of us through this delivery, the world had changed for the better.

Chapter 7

Healing from Loss

*There is a formidable though unconscious fear in our culture
that looking back at one's losses, failures or disappointments
will condemn one to eternal sorrow. . . . Facing loss directly
allows us to let go of the past and genuinely move on, in a way
that refusing to look back never does.*

Kim Kluger-Bell
*Unspeakable Losses: Understanding the Experience
of Pregnancy Loss, Miscarriage, and Abortion*
1998, p. 124

The period of pregnancy through postpartum presents a unique
opportunity for a woman to heal her past losses because it is a time
when feelings of grief pertaining to painful issues may surface. Traumatic experiences, whether during childhood, adolescence, or adult-
hood, may affect the pregnancy, birth, or the postpartum period. The
memory of significant losses may resurface in upsetting and distressing
ways as a woman enters motherhood.

WORKING WITH CLIENTS
DURING THE POSTPARTUM PERIOD

Working with women on issues of grief, loss, and fear prior to and
during pregnancy and the postpartum period is a central focus of my
practice. In addition to counseling women who have given birth by
cesarean section, I also counsel women who have experienced other
types of medical interventions such as the unwanted use of Pitocin or
episiotomy. Women who have experienced one or more miscarriages
or are dealing with the emotional issues of infertility also need sup-

port with their grieving processes. Other reproductive losses that present healing opportunities for pregnant women include later fetal demise, elective abortion, premature birth, release to adoption, birth of a seriously ill baby, stillbirth, or losing a baby to sudden infant death syndrome (SIDS).

Those who have experienced an early death of a mother, father, or sibling; have grown up in a family with a substance abuser; or have endured a history of abuse may be in need of specialized support. Any of these situations may evoke disturbing memories during pregnancy or postpartum that could compromise the woman's emotional and physical well-being. Some childbirth professionals may not be trained to deal with a client's history of abuse, loss, or trauma. They will refer a client to a qualified mental health provider. It is important to discuss this type of referral with the individual to help determine with whom she would feel most comfortable.

A woman who has experienced sexual, physical, or emotional abuse at any time in her life may face feelings of loss and sorrow during pregnancy or after giving birth. Tragically, many women have been physically or sexually abused or have witnessed abuse (Bass and Davis, 1988; Northrup, 1994; Pipher, 1994). It is estimated that one in three girls is sexually assaulted by the time she reaches age eighteen (Bass and Davis, 1988).

Women who present with issues of loss need to be attended to with gentle assistance. Acknowledging and validating the emotional distress of a woman's difficult memories is critical. Listening and empathizing with all of the life experiences a woman shares is an important aspect of the healing. In *The Courage to Heal,* Ellen Bass writes about working with survivors of sexual abuse, "The opportunity to be part of women's healing feels a little like assisting at a birth" (Bass and Davis, 1988, p. 15). This has also been my experience.

A pregnant woman may question the need to process past losses, which may be a challenging endeavor, at a time when she already feels physically and psychologically vulnerable. Some women will not want to take the risk of opening up this "can of worms" for fear of the strong feelings or memories that may be evoked. Once started, they may not want to complete the emotional journey. While working with my clients, I am often reminded that this healing work takes a great deal of courage and may not be for everyone. My hope is that the support a woman receives will enable her to move on through her pain to a place of satisfaction and contentment.

In the case of an individual who presents with any one of the losses I mention above, the childbirth professional's job is to listen to her, acknowledge her fear and pain, and allow her a safe place to feel her emotions. Some of my clients report that our sessions help them feel less isolated and lower their level of anxiety. Pregnant women deserve support and the opportunity to experience their emotions fully and process their past experiences to begin to feel some resolution.

Women have different levels of awareness about the emotional effects of their birth experiences. A woman who has had a difficult birth experience will often tell me that, since her baby is healthy, she has "nothing to complain about, no reason to talk." She may feel that she is not entitled to express feelings about her birthing experience. We discuss the fact that, while she is grateful for giving birth to a healthy baby, she also has experienced a major life transition, the exploration of which can be a profound and often therapeutic experience.

After giving birth, while a mother feels joy at the birth of a healthy baby, she may also experience a grief reaction, a profound sense of sadness as she adjusts to her new life as a parent. This reaction may arise when the birth did not go as she had hoped or expected. It may have to do with the ending of the pregnancy and the special connection she felt with the baby in her womb. In today's society, the woman may grieve the change in her identity from an independent working woman to one of the primary caregivers of a newborn. Upon returning to work after her maternity leave, another level of sadness may emerge as she leaves her baby in the care of others. The new mother's experience is affirmed when she is assured that she may have a wide range of emotions.

It is important for the childbirth professional to have done her own healing work and resolved some of her personal issues. Cathy Romeo and Claudia Panuthos discuss the many ways women can be helped to heal through reproductive losses in *Ended Beginnings*. The authors believe, "It is our task to heal ourselves so that these losses and this mourning process can become a rich source of blessings rather than unproductive suffering . . . we can be healed" (Panuthos and Romeo, 1984, p. 29). This is an important message for all of those who are working with pregnant and postpartum women.

Fay's Story: Multiple Losses

Fay came to me during her pregnancy to prepare individually for a VBAC. At our first session she talked about a number of losses that had occurred in her life. Her first pregnancy, prior to her cesarean birth, had ended in a miscarriage during the first trimester. Her grandmother had died several weeks after her miscarriage. In addition, when Fay was a teenager, a close family member experienced a stillbirth. Though this relative went on to later give birth to a healthy baby, Fay noted that the stillbirth had had a profound effect on her.

These major losses affected Fay's own experience of pregnancy and childbirth. She was "devastated" about her miscarriage, even after she attended a miscarriage support group that helped her deal with her sadness. She had been dismayed by the lack of understanding in our culture for this type of loss. Well-intentioned statements such as, "it was for the best" or "you will get pregnant again" made her feel alone. She felt that no one could understand why she was still so depressed a few months after the pregnancy loss. She became pregnant again within a few months of the miscarriage.

Fay's first full-term pregnancy continued with no signs of labor two and a half weeks past her due date. She confided that she had had a peculiar feeling for that entire pregnancy that she might not go into labor. She believed she held on to the pregnancy because she knew that "at least the baby was okay inside of me, but I did not know if he would be okay once he was born."

Fay had a great deal of fear about the physical pain of labor and birth. She did not go into labor and was induced by her obstetrician with Pitocin. After receiving Pitocin for about twelve hours, she had dilated to two centimeters. She was in a tremendous amount of pain and was given pain relief medication. She was told that the baby's position was high in the uterus, and that he had not descended into the correct position for a vaginal birth. Her obstetrician then suggested that she have a cesarean section. She agreed to the cesarean, and soon delivered a healthy baby boy.

With her VBAC labor, Fay began having contractions ten days past her due date. She told me she had a "rocky road" of labor for one day, with no dilation. After laboring for many hours with little progress, her midwife suggested starting Pitocin. Fay discussed this option with her midwife and felt satisfied because she participated in making the decision whether to use the labor-inducing medication. After five hours of Pitocin, Fay dilated to ten centimeters and was able to push. Fay gave birth vaginally to her baby girl. She later told me, "It was hard getting into effective labor. Then I was finally able to do it and everything went fine." Fay was delighted with her experience.

Donna's Story: Postpartum Adjustment

Donna scheduled an appointment with me when her second child, Todd, was almost one year old and her daughter, Marie, was a toddler. During our first appointment, Donna said that she was feeling overwhelmed by raising two young children and felt inadequate because her mother had raised more children "without complaining." Todd was a demanding baby, needing a great deal of her attention. Donna's husband was busy and tired much of the time. Her mother was also not available to help out with the new baby.

Although Donna stopped working at the end of her pregnancy, she kept Marie in day care two days a week. After Todd's birth, Donna was surprised at how much she missed her job. She longed for the interaction with adults and missed the challenge of accomplishing tasks. She had enjoyed and needed the monetary compensation.

I assured Donna that some of her feelings are those of loss; loss of her time and her old life, changes in the relationship with her husband, and loss of her identity as a working woman. There is so little support in our culture for women to comfortably experience feelings of loss after a normal healthy birth. Given the high percentage of working mothers, those who decide to stay home to raise their children may feel isolated caring for youngsters all day, when they were accustomed to being out in the working world with their peers. They often receive little help from extended family or other types of support systems.

At her next appointment, Donna told me about her childbirth experiences. Her daughter, Marie, was born by cesarean section eleven days past her due date. Her doctor had estimated the newborn's weight, according to the ultrasound, to be eight and one-half pounds. Instead, Marie weighed ten pounds at birth.

Because Marie was a large full-term baby, the obstetrician suggested that for the second baby, Donna be induced during her thirty-eighth week. Donna agreed to do this. While her obstetrician estimated the second baby's weight to be eight and one-half pounds, Todd weighed only six pounds six ounces. Donna felt very guilty about agreeing to be induced before her baby was full-term. She questioned whether the baby's medical problems, jaundice and colic, were her fault. In addition, she found her episiotomy to be very painful, "almost as bad as having a cesarean."

Donna had made the decision to be induced based on the explicit advice and information provided by her doctor, whom she had trusted. She felt anguish and great disappointment about her second birth experience. She blamed herself for following the unsound recommendation she had received. I asked her if she could forgive herself for agreeing to the early induction.

Donna was struggling with her daily life, suffering a sense of isolation and rejection from those she had hoped would support her. She felt alone and unable to accomplish routine household tasks. She had been efficient at completing assignments at work, but was now unable to take a shower in the morning or finish simple chores throughout the day. I suggested that she try to do something just for herself each day, such as taking a few moments to sit still, meditate, read, or take a bath. She needed to allow herself some time for self-care and self-love. Being part of a postpartum group, a circle of women where she could gain support and connect with other women in similar circumstances, would be beneficial for her. Confirmation that her feelings of guilt, loss, and isolation were natural was important for this client to begin to accept herself and work through her disappointment and sadness. She required some time to adjust to her role as a full-time mother of two children. I suggested that she be kind and patient with herself as she adapted to life at home.

A new mother deserves to be treated lovingly and with gentleness. If she wants to talk, those close to her should listen. She needs to feel supported, her role valued.

Fiona Shaw tells the horrifying story of her personal experience with postpartum depression, which began ten days after the birth of her second child, in her book, *Composing Myself: A Journey Through Postpartum Depression* (1998). As she slipped into serious debilitation, she wrote, "I longed for someone to take over, for someone, somehow, to mother me" (p. 26). After entering the hospital, during the first evening of her two-month hospitalization, Shaw questioned repeatedly, "I talked for hours. . . . Why couldn't I stop crying?" (p. 34). Upon reflection after her illness, Shaw wrote, "Both the talking and the writing have been vital to my recovery. . . . Somebody told me that not remembering much of this time would be a blessing. They were wrong" (p. 35). In my work with women, it is the remembering and telling of their stories that begins the healing process.

Chapter 8

Healing from Mother Loss

Pregnancy and the postpartum period can be bittersweet times for the motherless daughter, who feels closer to her mother as she becomes one but also feels an intense sadness as she confronts her loss again.

.

Hope Edelman
Motherless Daughters
1994, p. 246

COUNSELING MOTHERLESS WOMEN

A group of women whom I counsel are those whose mothers have died early in their lives. Early mother loss has a tremendous impact on a woman's life as she reaches the developmental milestone of becoming a mother herself. She may feel sorrow for the loss of her mother especially keenly during pregnancy or after giving birth. Her grief may resurface in disturbing and painful ways. It is very important for a woman who has suffered the premature death of her mother to connect with and gain specialized support from other women during pregnancy and the postpartum period.

The motherless woman may feel intensely alone and lost without the guidance of her own mother at this time. A pregnant woman whose mother has abandoned her, has been incarcerated, or was unavailable to her for other reasons might be in a situation similar to that of a woman whose mother is deceased. For women who feel that they were not mothered in the way they needed or would have wished, issues of unresolved loss can arise similar to those of women whose mothers have died.

Motherless Daughters, the landmark book on this subject by Hope Edelman (1994), explores the many consequences premature mother loss may have for a woman's life. Though a woman may feel that she has adequately grieved her mother's death, she becomes more vulnerable as she approaches the developmental stage of motherhood. "When a woman hasn't grieved her loss before pregnancy, she needs the safety to release any feelings that surface during that time without being made to feel overly needy and weak" (p. 246). She struggles with how to incorporate the loss of her mother into the next major adjustment of becoming a mother herself. For those who do not address this grief, it is possible that there may be a crisis during the birth or the postpartum period.

Psychologist Evelyn Bassoff writes in *Mothering Ourselves* (1991), "A woman who as a young child was insufficiently mothered can never fully make up what she missed. . . . [If] we take a chance and open ourselves up just a bit, we may find that others understand our loss and that in being understood we are somehow soothed" (p. 59). By having a chance to process her losses during pregnancy, by opening up and being understood, a woman prepares for the task of birthing and mothering her own child.

While working with motherless women during pregnancy, I help them revisit their grief and sadness and gently encourage them to feel their emotions. Coming to terms with the death of the mother can enable the woman to surrender to the incredible sensations that birth imposes on her. Women who have lost a mother at a young age continue to grieve that pain for a lifetime. But as these women approach the childbirth experience, the sadness that still exists for them as a result of mother loss may well be heightened. The grief may be confusing, and during childbirth, the labor may be slow or may stop. A woman's body may want to keep the baby inside her uterus where it is accustomed to being, where the outside world cannot harm it, the way the mother was harmed. A motherless woman can be helped through this difficulty by being with kind, communicative, and experienced people during the pregnancy, labor, and birth, in order to feel safe enough to have her baby.

Motherless women may miss the love and support of their own mothers acutely as they become mothers themselves. It does not matter if the loss occurred during the past year or thirty years ago; it is important for a woman to know she has the opportunity to process her feelings of grief at this time. The grieving process is just that, a process. Her feelings may not surface all at once, but as they do it helps to know there is someone with whom she can share them, and that she need not be afraid to feel them. There is a relief that comes with allowing the sadness to emerge. Many of my clients have felt some resolution after doing this important work.

Sara's Story: Patience, Support, and Time

Sara, who was planning a homebirth for the birth of her first baby, was referred to me by her midwife. A health care professional, Sara was well-informed about natural childbirth. She came for her first appointment during her fifth month of pregnancy. I also assisted at her homebirth.

At the first session, we talked about Sara's pregnancy. She also told me that her mother had died of breast cancer when Sara was thirteen years old. Her mother had survived two mastectomies, having been sick for one year. Sara said that she and her mother had never said goodbye to each other. During much of that first visit, Sara cried. It was a powerful experience to be present with her as she shared her feelings of loss with me.

During another prenatal session, Sara told me that, because she was still a child at the time of her mother's death, she had not been given the opportunity to fully grieve for her mother. At the time Sara was preparing to get married, a time of major change in her life, she had processed more of her unresolved grief. During the session she experienced waves of sadness about her mother's premature death.

We met regularly during her pregnancy and talked about labor, letting go, and surrendering to the pain. Her recurrent sadness about her mother's early death surfaced during some of our sessions. I felt her grieving was part of a process of her letting go of more sorrow in order to prepare for the birth. I told her that her ability to feel her emotions was an important component for her to be ready to surrender to the powerful sensations of labor. We talked about the possibility of Sara missing her mother during labor. She said that if she was aware of that happening, she would tell me or her husband at that time.

During another session with Sara, we did a visualization exercise during which I described labor contractions. I reminded her that she would get support from everyone who was present at the birth. When I talked about the possibility of her husband assisting her in the shower during labor, she cried. After the exercise, she said her mother was never able to ask anyone for help. While crying, she spoke about being happy that she is able to ask for help when she needs it. She asks for and receives assistance. She cried about her mother's inability to request support, and added that she would ask God for help to be with her in labor. Sara cried while she described a dream she had had, during which she gave birth to her baby and later her husband deserted her. Fear of abandonment can be especially present for a motherless pregnant woman. Edelman writes,

> Nearly every pregnant woman feels some anxiety about losing her partner and being left to parent a child alone, but this fear can become especially pronounced in a motherless woman. She knows all too well that people she loves can leave, and she remembers what happened to the last person she depended on to such a degree. (Edelman, 1994, p. 247)

During a prenatal visit, Sara told me that after her mom died, she and her siblings would go home from school and nap many afternoons. She realized that over the years, when things got rough for her, she would go to sleep.

We had planned for me to attend the homebirth, so Sara called me when it was time. When I arrived, the midwives were present and labor was progressing quickly. Sara's labor continued to advance and then slowed down at nine centimeters. She remained at this dilation for many hours, throughout the night and into the next day. There was concern that, if the labor did not proceed, Sara might need to be transported to the hospital.

It was suggested that Sara sit in a warm bath to help the labor progress. I sat on the edge of the tub talking with her for two hours. While we talked, she kept nodding off to sleep and we explored her sleeping at this significant point of labor. We reflected on the possibility that, by sleeping, she was trying to escape from having the baby. If a motherless woman has become accustomed to dealing with her problems in a certain way over the years, she may revert to this coping style in labor.

I began to question whether this baby was going to be born at home the way Sara had planned and desired. We talked more about her feelings at this time. I asked if she thought she was able to let the baby come into the world and experience the joy of the birth while still being sad about her mother's death. Could she feel sorrow and joy at the same time? She cried and said she thought she could. I asked her if she was able to stay awake and finish the very difficult work of giving birth to her baby. She agreed that she was sleeping to escape and she affirmed her wish to give birth to her baby at home. I asked her if she could continue her connection with her mother, which I knew included grief, and also be open to experiencing the delight of a new life. She replied that she could try to do this. I also suggested she let herself find a spiritual connection with her mother and ask her to help her give birth to the baby. She cried a bit in response. After I left the bathroom, the midwife went in and spent a few more hours with her while Sara rested in the tub.

A number of hours later, Sara gave birth to a beautiful, healthy baby girl. The labor took thirty hours. Sara was supported during her childbirth experience by her husband, as well as by many women—three midwives and myself. The midwives respected her need to take adequate time to give birth to her baby. They never tried to rush her; rather they waited and were very patient and encouraging. It was a beautiful experience to be present as Sara was able to push her baby out into the world with the loving assistance of her husband and the compassionate, knowledgeable midwives, Sara's circle of women.

After Sara gave birth to her daughter, she sent me this note:

> There are not enough words to thank you for all your support, knowledge, insight, and kindness throughout my pregnancy, labor, and delivery. I'm so very happy that our paths crossed.

Christine's Story:
The Need for Mothering and Connection

Christine had been referred to me after her first baby, Michelle, was born prematurely by cesarean section due to preeclampsia during Christine's thirty-second week of pregnancy. The birth was traumatic and Michelle was hospitalized for the first month of her life. This was very stressful for Christine, who visited and nursed the baby every day.

Once Michelle was able to come home, Christine began to feel intense anxiety. During our first session, Christine told me about her mother's death. Her mother had died suddenly in a car accident when Christine was fourteen years old. Her mother had undergone emergency surgery and had been in a coma for seven days before dying.

I began to see Christine every week and slowly her stress and tension began to decrease. We discussed the early death of her mother, as well as the premature birth of her baby. I listened to her story, often saying very little. I suggested that she surrender to her feelings, just as a laboring woman must surrender to the pain of labor. I encouraged her to allow herself to feel her anxiety, to be aware of her feelings, and to tell herself, "I feel anxious; I surrender to this anxiety." Christine needed to be reassured that it is not unusual for a woman who is grieving her losses to be upset. She could allow herself to let her sadness emerge. I also affirmed that being a new mother is a demanding job.

Months later, during a session, I asked Christine if she could accept that she is in an uncomfortable position right now with all of her awareness and concerns. Could she acknowledge that she was exactly where she was supposed to be in her process? This question calmed her. I suggested she accept herself and not blame herself for the birth. I wanted her to know that the birth took place the way it did for a reason, a reason we will probably never know. Christine shared with me that she had a sense her mother was watching over her.

During the course of Christine's counseling, she became pregnant for the second time and we continued with our work. She knew she needed the support of a woman to discuss her feelings and worries about pregnancy and her ability to be a mother. Christine found meditation and visualization exercises to be calming and we often utilized them during a session. The practice, at times, would be to sit, breathe, and relax. At other times, after having her relax, I would speak to Christine about visualizing a safe, quiet place for her to see herself resting peacefully.

When she was in the tenth week of her second pregnancy, Christine spoke about hearing the baby's heartbeat for the first time at her prenatal appointment. She felt sadness that her mother was not alive to share this experience. A few days later, she experienced severe pain in her abdomen, followed by brown spotting. Christine was "devastated that her baby may not be okay." The doctor reassured her that everything was fine, but that she should rest.

During the session after the spotting incident, I suggested we do a meditation about the healthy growth and development of her second baby. She sobbed when I told her she was helping her baby grow in just the right way. After this meditation, she related that she realized she could not protect her baby; she could only do so much. She said that during this meditation exercise she had visualized a disturbing memory of her mother's casket being lowered into the ground. She realized upon seeing this image that she had not been able to save her mother and remembered feeling all alone during the time of her mother's death. She cried in the session and said she had never before allowed herself to cry so much. I told her she was doing a wonderful job taking care of herself and the growing baby inside of her. I recognized her for doing the challenging work of permitting the grief to emerge. I encouraged her to take care of herself and write in her journal while continuing this healing process.

During the twenty-third week of her pregnancy, Christine experienced the sixteenth anniversary of her mother's death and visited the grave site. While in the cemetery, though she felt sad, Christine noted that she was impressed by the beauty of the flowers, the sun, and the feeling of life all around her. She thought of her mother as a resource to help her through her struggles. She imagined herself gaining strength from the memory of her mother. This connection with her mother helped her through the difficult moments of anxiety and sadness.

The following week, Christine began to have Braxton Hicks contractions, a common occurrence during the second trimester. These contractions, though not painful, reminded her of the early labor she had experienced with her first pregnancy, resulting in the traumatic premature birth of Michelle. Christine was extremely anxious and was seen by her doctor. She said, "It [the appointment] felt a little crisis-like. In order to go to the hospital I needed to get someone to come care for Michelle." After being checked and assured that she was fine, she felt relieved and went home. The doctor suggested she rest if she was having more than four contractions per hour.

She cried as she told me she was ". . . feeling tested. I don't want to repeat this pattern. How can I get through this without it turning into a crisis?" I acknowledged that having the sensation of contractions was difficult because the contractions reminded her of the first traumatic birth. I asked her if she was able to separate the two pregnancies while she prepared to have the second baby. I told her I believed that she could remain in spiritual connection with her mother without a crisis, that she deserved to have a healthy pregnancy and a peaceful birth.

For Christine, nearing her thirty-second week of pregnancy was a milestone because of Michelle's birth at thirty-two weeks. She had not wanted to discuss preparing for a vaginal birth after cesarean (VBAC) with me or her obstetrician until reaching this point in her pregnancy. Now we were able to begin to explore the various issues involved in planning for a VBAC.

The day before our appointment, during Christine's thirty-first week of pregnancy, she had seen her obstetrician, who had informed her of the very rare possibility of uterine rupture with a VBAC. During our session she sobbed, remembering the impact of the doctor's use of the word "rupture." This language had triggered Christine's memories of her mother's emergency surgery and death, and her own fears about death. She had associated all of her mother's limbs coming apart and rupturing with the mention of the word "rupture." I listened and then told her that, though her first birth with its emergency surgery may have connected her to her mother, who had emergency surgery after her accident, it was quite unlikely that another situation would happen like that again.

We briefly discussed her doctor's insistence on the use of an IV "in case of an emergency," because she was a VBAC candidate. I suggested that an IV was not necessary if she drank fluids during labor and that it might be a setup for further medical intervention. A healthy pregnant woman, VBAC or not, only requires an IV if she has been in the hospital for many hours without eating or drinking and is becoming dehydrated, or has the need for pain medication or Pitocin. I hoped that we could talk about this further as the pregnancy progressed.

Christine voiced her concern about getting stuck during dilation. I explained that this is a common fear for VBAC women. Utilizing guidelines, such as not going to the hospital too early, resting, eating, and drinking fluids during labor are important ways for a woman to empower herself at that time. We planned to discuss these details further in the next weeks.

This was a significant session for Christine and for me. She later wrote in her journal:

> It started to surface when I asked Dr. M. yesterday how much monitoring would take place at the birth if everything went smoothly. She said the main thing would be having an IV, because of my previous c-section, but I could still move around, take a shower, etc. I asked why an IV and she said in the extremely unlikely event that the scar ruptures (1/10,000), and they had to do emergency surgery, they wouldn't want to play around putting an IV in. That tapped into a lot for me.
>
> Here I had been feeling so positive lately, I am almost 32 weeks, and made it over this huge hurdle, and have worked so hard to get to this place and feel good. And now, here was one more thing thrown in my face stirring up the "something bad could happen" anxiety—yes it's incredibly unlikely, but so was my mom's death. Here I pictured myself home free, and now there's another emotional hurdle right at the very end.
>
> Then there's the whole connection with my mother having emergency surgery, this image of them bringing her in, and not being able to fix her, to make her all better.
>
> When I talked about that with Lois, I totally lost it and began sobbing uncontrollably. It hit upon this very deep, buried grief and pain. And then there's the connection with my own emergency surgery at Michelle's birth, and that whole crisis and the fear that evokes.
>
> Lois' initial reaction to the IV was that it treats a healthy pregnant woman like a "sick" patient, waiting for an emergency to happen. For some reason, that whole thing symbolized for me again this sense of no guarantees, so I won't get pre-eclampsia, but that doesn't promise nothing else bad will happen. It calls upon this profound sense of trust to be able to allow myself to do this birth, when a scared part of myself wonders, can I really do this? This is so hard—
>
> Also, the whole image of the scar rupturing represented symbolically this image of all my terrible pain and grief and sadness about my mom just erupting—as if it's all down there

somewhere and all of that pain I'm not often in touch with could well up and overwhelm me. When I talked to Lois about that I also sobbed uncontrollably.

Christine went swimming, an activity that she generally found relaxing and enjoyable. While swimming, she was seized by a sense of fear. She went home and decided to sit down and try to stay with her feelings, as I had encouraged her to do in the past. She meditated, bringing her focus to her breathing while remaining present with the fear. She later continued writing in her journal:

> When I was swimming, I was thinking about this basic human fear I am connected to—this raw fear that is part of me, that is probably the hardest emotion to let myself acknowledge—that is pushed down the deepest. I am sure I felt it around the time of my mother's accident—but I was in such shock that I became numb to it, couldn't really process it (it was much too threatening). This *fear* of losing my *mother,* the central person in my life, the person who took care of me and nurtured me—what would be left of my world without her, who would take care of me in that special way?—fear of abandonment, of being left alone. . . . And I know that fear must have surfaced during Michelle's birth, but again I couldn't process it—fear of my own mortality, vulnerability, fragility of life.
>
> I was thinking that maybe part of what is getting tapped into has to do with accepting this place of fear in me, facing it, giving it existence—and by allowing myself to be in that space, that part of myself and my experience, to somehow find strength in that. There was also an image I had of being a scared little girl and going back in time to acknowledge that.
>
> Again, this all brings me in touch with my deepest fears—of not having *control* over bad things, of not having a guarantee in life that everything will be 100 percent okay, of not having control over my own mortality or those I love.

During the thirty-seventh week of the pregnancy, Christine's baby was found to be in the breech position. The doctor suggested an external version, a procedure to try to turn the baby to a head-down position. Christine was disappointed when her obstetrician informed her that if the version did not work, a cesarean section would be necessary to deliver the baby. Her obstetrician attempted the external version but it was not successful in changing the baby's position. She was then scheduled for a cesarean section to be performed during her thirty-ninth week. We discussed the alternative of waiting to have the cesarean after labor had begun because contractions help stimulate the baby's lungs for breathing. She decided to proceed with the scheduled cesarean and not wait for labor to begin. We discussed having the support of her labor assistant during the cesarean. She decided she wanted her labor assistant to stay with her and her husband during the cesarean.

A few days before her scheduled cesarean, Christine had a session with me followed by one with her body work practitioner. That evening, she spontaneously went into labor. She and her husband went to the hospital where they met their labor assistant, who stayed with them during the cesarean section. She had dilated to three centimeters before having the cesarean. In addition to being with her before and during the operation, the labor assistant stayed in Christine's room with her the entire first night of the baby's life, while her husband went home to be with their older child. This enabled Christine to keep her baby in the room with her. After her first cesarean, Christine had not held her baby until many hours after the birth. She was very grateful to her labor assistant for all of her support.

Although Christine did not have the vaginal birth that she had hoped for, she found her second cesarean to be a satisfying, fulfilling experience. She had begun labor without medical intervention and then had an uncomplicated cesarean and a full-term healthy baby. During this pregnancy and birth Christine had met helpful, supportive women with whom she stayed in contact on a regular basis. Her yoga instructor (who also was her body work practitioner), her labor assistant, her child care provider, and I supported her through this period. She had found the mothering she needed. Two weeks after her second cesarean, Christine felt "centered and content."

Christine wrote a note to me after the birth of her son:

> The work I did with you during my pregnancy . . . has been incredibly powerful for me. I can't imagine what my experience would have been like had I not been working with you—I am

only grateful for all of your help which enabled me to grow emotionally and spiritually, and which played such an important part in bringing my beautiful son into the world.

You have been such a source of support for me, and have helped me discover my own inner strengths and resources. The grief work around my mother's death has ultimately helped me feel more connected with her. And I am beginning to know an inner peace I had not known before.

A motherless woman can experience profound healing during pregnancy and childbirth by accessing help from her circle of women, her partner, and spiritual guidance from her mother. Both Sara and Christine gained courage through these connections.

PART V:
BIRTH AS A SACRED
EXPERIENCE

Chapter 9

Circle of Women

The family, or people who are close to the person who is in the passage of being born or who is leaving, need to have what I would call sacred space. They need to be protected from insensitive people, from intrusions by people who don't know what is going on. They need to have their needs seen to, even if they are not able to articulate them themselves. . . . Sacred space isn't so much physical space, although it may be, it's the emotional and spiritual space.

Ina May Gaskin
in Penfield Chester, *Sisters on a Journey*
1997, p. 133

Throughout this book I have spoken about the meaningfulness of women supporting one another during pregnancy, childbirth, and postpartum. Creating a circle of support helps a woman have a fulfilling childbirth experience. This circle consists of the woman and her partner, a childbirth educator, a midwife or physician, a labor assistant, and other pregnant women. Supportive friends and family as well as body work practitioners can also play significant roles. The emotional and physical assistance men provide is crucial. In this model of childbirth preparation, women become empowered to know who they want in their circle, find them, and enlist their help. Sometimes women have accessed support from their ancestors. Giving birth should be approached as a sacred experience by the birthing woman as well as those who assist her.

A woman deserves to have a fulfilling childbirth experience. Painful occurrences such as a previous traumatic birth, premature death of a close family member, miscarriage, or other loss may profoundly affect the upcoming birth. Pregnancy and the postpartum time present a unique opportunity for her to speak about her life in order to prepare for the birth of her baby. She may wish to speak to any one of the members of her support circle. Sharing her feelings about past losses, and concerns about the birth and parenting is reassuring. The individualized attention, knowing that she has a listener who is present for her, can increase her confidence in her own abilities.

Ina May Gaskin talks about the similarity between the energy of birth and the energy of death. My work with a motherless woman as she grieves the death of her mother asserts that the intensity of working through this pain is valuable. Gaskin's reference to a "sacred space" for pregnant women describes the life-affirming peace and support that Christine, the motherless woman in Chapter 8, discovered after spending time during her visualization in her special place.

Christine and I had practiced meditation and visualization in our sessions. During her second pregnancy, she was feeling a lack of control over her life and an absence of safety in the world. Christine was able to enter the following meditation while remaining with her terror. By imagining this vision, she gained peace and serenity. Her image of a circle of women helped her cope with the early death of her mother and empowered her for her second birth experience and for her life:

> . . . I just did a meditation to try and connect with the space of fear in me. I start off in my inner sanctuary, a place of safety. But then I venture out into the woods, into the darkness. I am alone, lost, afraid—afraid of the wild animals, of being attacked or eaten alive. I guess afraid of the unknown (that I cannot see). As I keep wandering deeper in the woods I come across a group of (primitive, tribal) women, gathered around a big fire, all in a circle, dancing. They each have their faces painted—they are chanting as they dance. I am surrounded by these women, in the middle of the circle—and in all its pain I give birth—I begin to push the baby out, just there by myself (as I imagine primitive women must have done, with no interventions). As the head crowns, one of the women comes up and holds the head, catching and cradling the baby as it comes out. She hands the baby to me and I put it to my breast, and the baby nurses. I look up and recognize the familiar face of my mother for a moment (beneath the face paint) as the one standing with me, who held the baby for a moment before giving it to me. But when I look for her again, she has

already disappeared within the circle of women, and I cannot find her. (Although I cannot have her in my life, I know her spirit is with me.)

Christine found this image of her mother within the circle of women inspiring and soothing. Though she did not go on to the have the birth she had hoped for, she was content with her childbirth and immediate postpartum experience, having processed a great deal of sadness and fear while finding the nurturing support she needed.

COMPASSIONATE CHILDBIRTH PREPARATION

Elisabeth Kübler-Ross (1997) wrote, "I think modern medicine has become like a prophet offering a life free of pain. It is nonsense. The only thing I know that truly heals people is unconditional love" (p. 15). Being compassionate and reassuring is of primary significance in the way that I work with women. I have the feeling in my heart of deeply caring about women and their experiences of giving birth. By allowing a woman the sacred space to speak about her pregnancy, birth, and postpartum adjustment, she receives the support and encouragement she deserves as she proceeds through these major life transitions.

My work in helping women endure and heal from their grief and sadness connects me to the memory of my ancestors. One of my circles of women includes my relatives. My grandmothers and their mothers are included in the circle with my own immediate family. Sadie, my mother's mother, and Sarah, my father's mother, both became motherless at five years of age. I do not have any information about my grandmother Sarah's mother. Sadie's mother died while giving birth. Her grandmother died when Sadie, then just a teenager, was planning her wedding. Two occasions that are usually associated with joy, a birth and a wedding, were shrouded in death and sorrow. I feel a strong connection with the women of my family who suffered their losses in silence, with little or no support. Though their voices were not heard, I am able to speak for them.

Within the circle of relatives are my children, who are both teenagers now. My son Scott is named for my two grandmothers, his great-grandmothers. His traumatic birth was the impetus for my pursuing a VBAC and sent me on a journey of self-reflection and change. Preparing for the VBAC inspired me to explore my inner resources and discover a part of myself that was strong, assertive, and passionate. The birth of my daughter Melissa changed my life. It motivated me to seek my chosen career of counseling women and couples during and after pregnancy. I am honored to support women and their partners, all within the circle, as they advocate for their births and make important choices for their lives.

Just as a woman's children are part of her legacy to the world, so are the stories of her pregnancies and births. These stories often illustrate the struggle inherent in the birthing process. They also catalog the innate strength that I believe all women possess. When women are given the tools, support, and encouragement that they need, many find incredible reserves of energy and power to birth their babies and find the joy in their experiences.

All of the women in this book exhibited great strength. Christine's story is one of courage. She was able to confront her fears and process her grief while preparing for her second birth. Christine was helped by the spiritual presence of the circle of women in her meditation and by the women who supported her during the pregnancy and birth. She writes of the hope she found in her meditation after birthing her baby within the sacred circle of women:

> . . . I carry the baby back through the woods to my sanctuary, and sit with the baby in the pool of water I often imagine there, with a small waterfall overhead.
>
> Before I began on this journey to confront my fears, I imagined in doing so that I might find something to bring home with me that would give me strength and courage. I realize, as I sit in the water, that it is the baby—this new life emerging in spite of any fears or unknowns or loss—this sense of life going on, the chain continuing, in spite of anything scary or tragic or sad—that represents the ultimate faith, the ultimate trust—the courage to go on despite anything else.

I have gained strength from many circles of women in my life. As I planned for my second birth, I was inspired and encouraged by Nancy Cohen and the couples in the VBAC preparation series she led.

Women shared their experience of VBAC with me during that pregnancy. My compassionate labor assistant supported me within my circle. She gave me the encouragement and confidence to achieve my goal of a vaginal birth. Later, I met Miriam Greenspan and the circle of women she assembled. My journey of self-reflection continued.

My circle of women extends to my individual clients and the prenatal and postpartum groups I have led. Both women and men have shared their stories with me and allowed me to be part of their healing. These special people have taught me the value of compassionate support again and again. I am grateful and honored to have been given the chance to be part of their childbirth experiences and their lives.

It has taken another circle of women and men to support me in telling my story and those of my clients. My family, friends, colleagues, and other healers have coached me through the natural birthing process of this book and have patiently assisted as the words have found their way out of my heart and onto paper. I am so grateful to all of them. My hope is that the stories in this book encourage women to acknowledge and speak about their experiences of loss, pregnancy, childbirth, and postpartum. There are many more stories in all of the women I know, waiting to be heard. In this way, the process of growth, change, and healing continues.

Bibliography

Affonso, D. (1977). Missing pieces—a study of postpartum feelings. *Birth and the Family Journal 4*(4), 159-164.

Affonso, D.D. and Stichler, J.F. (1978). Exploratory study of women's reactions to having a cesarean birth. *Birth and the Family Journal 5*(2), 88-94.

Arms, S. (1975). *Immaculate Deception*. Boston: Houghton Mifflin.

Armstrong, P. and Feldman, S. (1990). *A Wise Birth*. New York: William Morrow and Co., Inc.

Baldwin, R. (1986). *Special Delivery*. Berkeley, CA: Celestial Arts.

Ballinger, C.B. (1982). Emotional disturbance during pregnancy and following delivery. *Journal of Psychosomatic Research 26*(6), 629-634.

Bass, E. and Davis, L. (1988). *The Courage to Heal*. New York: Harper & Row.

Bassoff, E. (1991). *Mothering Ourselves: Help and Healing for Adult Daughters*. New York: Dutton, Penguin Books.

Belenky, M.F., Clinchy, B.M., Goldberger, N.R., and Tarule, J.M. (1986). *Women's Ways of Knowing: The Development of Self, Voice, and Mind*. New York: Basic Books, Inc.

Blonski, M. (1989). Teaching about the influence of the environment on the birthing process. *International Journal of Childbirth Education 4*(1), 32-33.

Bloom, S.L., McIntire, D.D., Kelly, M., Beimer, H.L., Burpo, R.H., Garcia, M.A., and Leveno, K.J. (1998). Lack of effect of walking on labor and delivery. *The New England Journal of Medicine 339*(2), 76-79.

Borysenko, J. (1990). *Guilt Is the Teacher, Love Is the Lesson*. New York: Warner Books, Inc.

The Boston Women's Health Book Collective, Inc. (1970). *Our Bodies, Ourselves: A Book By and For Women*. Somerville, MA: New England Free Press.

Bradley, C.F., Ross, S.E., and Warnyca, J. (1983). A prospective study of mothers' attitudes and feelings following cesarean and vaginal births. *Birth 10*(2), 79-83.

Brewer, G. (1978). *The Pregnancy-After-30 Workbook*. Emmaus, PA: Rodale Press.

Brewer, G. and Greene, J.P. (1981). *Right from the Start*. Emmaus, PA: Rodale Press.

Chester, P. (1997). *Sisters on a Journey: Portraits of American Midwives*. New Brunswick, NJ: Rutgers University Press.

Clark, C. (1987). Vaginal birth after cesarean section. *International Journal of Childbirth Education 2*(4), 21-27.

Clark, S.L. (1988). Rupture of the scarred uterus. *Obstetrics and Gynecology Clinics of North America 15*(4), 737-744.

Cohen, N.W. (1977). Minimizing emotional sequellae of cesarean childbirth. *Birth and the Family Journal 4*(3), 114-119.

Cohen, N. (1991). *Open Season: A Survival Guide for Natural Childbirth and VBAC in the 90's.* New York: Bergin and Garvey.

Cohen, N. and Estner, L. (1983). *Silent Knife: Cesarean Prevention and Vaginal Birth After Cesarean.* South Hadley, MA: Bergin and Garvey Publishers, Inc.

Conner, B. (1977). Teaching about cesarean birth in traditional childbirth classes. *Birth and the Family Journal 4*(3), 107-113.

Cragin, E.B. (1916). Conservatism in Obstetrics. *New York Medical Journal 104*(1), 1-3.

Cranley, M.S., Hedahl, K.J., and Pegg, S.H. (1983). Women's perceptions of vaginal and cesarean deliveries. *Nursing Research 32*(1), 10-14.

Crawford, K. (1990). A successful labor support service for VBAC families. *International Journal of Childbirth Education 5*(1), 36-37.

Crawford, K. and Walters, J. (1996). *Natural Childbirth After Cesarean.* Cambridge, MA: Blackwell Science, Inc.

Davis, E. (1987). *Heart and Hands: A Midwife's Guide to Pregnancy and Birth.* Berkely, CA: Celestial Arts.

Debrovner, C.H. and Shubin, R. (1985). Pregnancy and postpartum part 2: Postpartum sexual concerns. *Medical Aspects of Human Sexuality 19*(5), 84-90.

DeLee, J.B. (1920). The prophylactic forceps operation. *The American Journal of Obstetrics and Gynecology 1*(1), 34-44.

DiMatteo, M.R., Morton, S.C., Carney, M.F., Pearson, M., Lepper, H.S., Damush, T.M., and Kahn, K.L. (1996). Cesarean childbirth and psychosocial outcomes: A meta-analysis. *Health Psychology 15*(4), 303–314.

Edelman, H. (1994). *Motherless Daughters: The Legacy of Loss.* New York: Delta Books.

Edelman, H. (1995). *Letters from Motherless Daughters: Words of Courage, Grief, and Healing.* Reading, MA: Addison-Wesley Publishing Co.

Eggers, P. (1987). VBAC couples in refresher classes: Some solutions to the challenge. *International Journal of Childbirth Education 2*(3), 32-33.

Ehrenreich, B. and English, D. (1973). *Witches, Midwives, and Nurses: A History of Women Healers.* New York: The Feminist Press.

Enkin, M. (1977). Having a section is having a baby. *Birth and the Family Journal 4*(3), 99-105.

Erb, L., Hill, G., and Houston, D. (1983). A survey of parents' attitudes toward their cesarean births in Manitoba hospitals. *Birth 10*(2), 85-91.

Flamm, B.L. (1990). *Birth After Cesarean.* New York: Simon & Schuster.

Flamm, B.L. and Goings, J.R. (1989). Vaginal birth after cesarean section: Is suspected fetal macrosomia a contraindication? *Obstetrics and Gynecology 74*(5), 694-697.

Galinsky, E. (1981). *Between Generations: The Six Stages of Parenthood.* New York: The New York Times Book Co., Inc.

Garel, M., Lelong, N., and Kaminski, M. (1987). Psychological consequences of caesarean childbirth in primiparas. *Journal of Psychosomatic Obstetrics and Gynecology 6*(3), 197-209.

Garel, M., Lelong, N., and Kaminski, M. (1988). Follow-up study of psychological consequences of caesarean childbirth. *Early Human Development 16*(2-3), 271-282.

Gaskin, I.M. (1978). *Spiritual Midwifery,* Revised Edition. Summertown, TN: Book Publishing Co.

Gilligan, C. (1982). *In a Different Voice: Psychological Theory and Women's Development.* Cambridge, MA: Harvard University Press.

Gottlieb, S. and Barrett, D. (1986). Effects of unanticipated cesarean section on mothers, infants, and their interaction in the first month of life. *Journal of Developmental and Behavioral Pediatrics 7*(3), 180-185.

Greene, G., Zeichner, A., Roberts, N.L., Callahan, E.J., and Granados, J.L. (1989). Preparation for cesarean delivery: A multicomponent analysis of treatment outcome. *Journal of Consulting and Clinical Psychology 57*(4), 484-487.

Greenspan, M. (1983). *A New Approach to Women and Therapy.* New York: McGraw-Hill.

Hart, G. (1980). Maternal attitudes in prepared and unprepared cesarean deliveries. *Journal of Obstetric, Gynecologic, and Neonatal Nursing 9*(4), 243-245.

Heinowitz, J. (1995). *Pregnant Fathers: Entering Parenthood Together.* San Diego, CA: Parents as Partners Press.

Herzfeld, J. (1985). *Sense and Sensibility in Childbirth.* New York: W.W. Norton & Co.

Jones, C. (1991). *The Expectant Parent's Guide to Preventing a Cesarean Section.* New York: Bergin and Garvey.

Jordan, B. (1987). The hut and the hospital: Information, power, and symbolism in the artifacts of birth. *Birth 14*(1), 36-40.

Jordan, J.V., Kaplan, A.G., Miller, J.B., Stiver, I.P., and Surrey, J.L. (1991). *Women's Growth in Connection.* New York: Guilford Press.

Jordan, J.V., Surrey, J.L., and Kaplan, A.G. (1991). Women and empathy: Implications for psychological development and psychotherapy. In J.V. Jordan, A.G. Kaplan, J.B. Miller, I.P Stiver, and J.L. Surrey, *Women's Growth in Connection,* pp. 27-50. New York: Guilford Press.

Kennell, J., Klaus, M., McGrath, S., Robertson, S., and Hinkley, C. (1991). Continuous emotional support during labor in a U.S. hospital: A randomized controlled trial. *Journal of the American Medical Association 265*(17), 2197-2201.

Kitzinger, S. (1984). *The Experience of Childbirth.* New York: Penguin Books.

Kitzinger, S. (1996). *The Complete Book of Pregnancy and Childbirth.* New York: Alfred A. Knopf, Inc.

Klaus, M., Kennell, J., Klaus, P. (1993). *Mothering the Mother.* Reading, MA: Addison-Wesley Publishing Co.

Kluger-Bell, K. (1998). *Unspeakable Losses: Understanding the Experience of Pregnancy Loss, Miscarriage, and Abortion.* New York: W.W. Norton & Co.

Knox, R. (1998). "Hospital drive is cutting rate of caesareans." *The Boston Globe,* September 21, pp. C1, C4.

Koehler, N. (1985). *Artemis Speaks: VBAC Stories and Natural Childbirth Information.* Occidental, CA: Jerald R. Brown, Inc.

Kort, C. and Friedland, R. (1986). *The Fathers' Book: Shared Experiences.* Boston: G. K. Hall & Co.

Korte, D. (1997). *The VBAC Companion: The Expectant Mother's Guide to Vaginal Birth After Cesarean.* Boston: Harvard Common Press.

Korte, D. and Scaer, R. (1984). *A Good Birth, a Safe Birth.* New York: Bantam Books.

Kübler-Ross, E. (1997). *The Wheel of Life: A Memoir of Living and Dying.* New York: Scribner.

Kushner, E. (1997). *Experiencing Abortion: A Weaving of Women's Words.* Binghamton, NY: Harrington Park Press.

Lewis, P. (1987). Therapeutic change in groups: An interactional perspective. *Small Group Behavior 18*(4), 548-556.

Lipson, J. (1981). Cesarean support groups: Mutual help and education. *Women and Health 6*(3/4), 27-39.

Litoff, J.B. (1978). *American Midwives: 1860 to the Present.* Westport, CT: Greenwood Press.

Llewelyn, S.P. and Haslett, A.V.J. (1986). Factors perceived as helpful by the members of self-help groups: An exploratory study. *British Journal of Guidance and Counseling 14*(3), 252-262.

Lomas, J., Enkin, M., Anderson, G., Hannah, W., Vayda, E., and Singer, J. (1991). Opinion leaders versus audit and feedback to implement practice guidelines: Delivery after previous cesarean section. *Journal of the American Medical Association 265*(17), 2202-2207.

Lumley, J. (1985). Assessing satisfaction with childbirth. *Birth 12*(3), 141-145.

MacDorman, M.F. and Singh, G. (1998). Midwifery care, social and medical risk factors and birth outcomes in the USA. *Journal of Epidemiology and Community Health 52*(5), 310-317.

Marut, J. and Mercer, R. (1979). Comparison of primiparas' perception of vaginal and cesarean births. *Nursing Research 28*(5), 260-266.

McMahon, M.J., Luther, E.R., Bowes, W.A. Jr., and Olshan, A.F. (1996). Comparison of a trial of labor with an elective second cesarean section. *New England Journal of Medicine, 335*(10), 689-695.

Miller, J.B. (1976). *Toward a New Psychology of Women.* Boston: Beacon Press.

Miller, J.B. and Stiver, I.P. (1997). *The Healing Connection: How Women Form Relationships in Therapy and in Life.* Boston: Beacon Press.

Morford, M. and Barclay, L. (1984). Counseling the pregnant woman: Implications for birth outcomes. *The Personnel and Guidance Journal 62*(10), 619-623.

Murphey, T. (1984). Encouraging client responsibility. *Individual Psychology Journal of Adlerian Theory, Research, and Practice 40*(2), 122-132.

Myers, S.A., and Gleicher, N. (1988). A successful program to lower cesarean section rates. *New England Journal of Medicine 319*(23), 1511-1516.

Nelson, M.K. (1981). Client responses to a discrepancy between the care they want and the care they receive. *Women and Health 6*(3/4), 135-152.

Northrup, C. (1994). *Women's Bodies, Women's Wisdom.* New York: Bantam Books.

Norwood, C. (1984). *How to Avoid a Cesarean Section.* New York: Simon and Schuster, Inc.

Norwood, C. (1986). Cesarean variation: Patients, facilities or policies. *International Journal of Childbirth Education 1*(3), 4, 14.

Novas, J., Myers, S.A., and Gleicher, N. (1989). Obstetric outcome of patients with more than one previous cesarean section. *American Journal of Obstetrics and Gynecology 160*(2), 364-367.

Osherson, S. (1986). *Finding Our Fathers: How a Man's Life Is Shaped by His Relationship with His Father.* New York: Fawcett Columbine.

Padawer, J.A., Fagan, C., Janoff-Bulman, R., Strickland, B.R., and Chorowshi, M. (1988). Women's psychological adjustment following emergency cesarean versus vaginal birth. *Psychology of Women Quarterly 12*(1), 25-34.

Panuthos, C. and Romeo, C. (1984). *Ended Beginnings: Healing Childbearing Losses.* South Hadley, MA: Bergin and Garvey Publishers, Inc.

Paul, R.H. (1996). Toward fewer cesarean sections—the role of a trial of labor. *New England Journal of Medicine 335*(10), 735-736.

Pearson, J. (1988). The phobic's experience of childbirth. *International Journal of Childbirth Education 3*, 44-45.

Perez, P.G. (1988). The emotional work of pregnancy. *International Journal of Childbirth Education 3*, 30-31.

Perez, P. and Snedeker, C. (1990). *Special Women: The Role of the Professional Labor Assistant.* Seattle, WA: Pennypress, Inc.

Peterson, G. (1981). *Birthing Normally.* Berkeley, CA: Mindbody Press.

Petitti, D. (1985). Recent trends in cesarean delivery rates in California. *Birth 12*(1), 25-28.

Phelan, J.F., Ahn, M.O., Diaz, F., Brar, H.S., and Rodriguez, M.H. (1989). Twice a cesarean, always a cesarean? *Obstetrics and Gynecology 73*(2), 161-165.

Pipher, M. (1994). *Reviving Ophelia: Saving the Selves of Adolescent Girls.* New York: Ballantine Books.

Poisson-Salomon, A.S., Breart, G., Maillard, F., Rabarison, Y., Chavigny, C., Sureau, C., and Rumeau-Roquette, C. (1986). Can the number of cesarean sections be reduced without risk? An analysis of rates and indications in a university clinic. *European Journal of Obstetrical and Gynecological Reproductive Biology 22*(5/6), 297-307.

Poole, C.M. and Parr, E.A. (1994). *Choosing a Nurse-Midwife: Your Guide to Safe, Sensitive Care During Pregnancy and the Birth of Your Child.* New York: John Wiley & Sons, Inc.

Porreco, R.P. (1985). High cesarean section rate: A new perspective. *Obstetrics and Gynecology 65*(3), 307-311.

Raphael, D. (1973). *The Tender Gift: Breastfeeding.* New York: Schocken Books.

Remen, R.N. (1996). *Kitchen Table Wisdom: Stories that Heal.* New York: Riverhead Books.

Rich, A. (1976). *Of Woman Born: Motherhood As Experience and Institution.* New York: W.W. Norton & Co., Inc.

Richards, L.B. (1987). *The Vaginal Birth After Cesarean Experience.* South Hadley, MA: Bergin and Garvey Publishers, Inc.

Richards, M.P.M. (1982). The trouble with "choice" in childbirth. *Birth 9*(4), 253-260.

Rothman, B.K. (1985). Beyond risks and rates in obstetric care. *Birth 12*(2), 91-94.

Rothman, B.K. (1986). *The Tentative Pregnancy: Prenatal Diagnosis and the Future of Motherhood.* New York: Viking Penguin.

Rothman, B.K. (1991). *In Labor: Women and Power in the Birthplace.* New York: W.W. Norton & Co., Inc.

Shapiro, J. (1987). *When Men Are Pregnant: Needs and Concerns of Expectant Fathers.* San Luis Obispo, CA: Impact Publishers.

Shaw, F. (1998). *Composing Myself: A Journey Through Postpartum Depression.* South Royalton, VT: Steerforth Press.

Simkin, P. (1989). Childbearing in social context. *Women and Health 15*(3), 5-21.

Simkin, P., Whalley, J., and Keppler, A. (1991). *Pregnancy, Childbirth and the Newborn.* New York: Meadowbrook Press.

Smith, J. (1992). *Women and Doctors.* New York: Monthly Press.

Stafford, R.S. (1990). Alternative strategies for controlling rising cesarean section rates. *Journal of the American Medical Association 263*(5), 683-687.

Sundin, J. (1988). The presence of pain. *International Journal of Childbirth Education 3*(3), 16-17.

Taffel, S.M., Placek, P.J., and Liss, T. (1987). Trends in the United States cesarean section rate and reasons for the 1980-1985 rise. *American Journal of Public Health 77*(8), 955-959.

Yalom, I.D. and Vinogradov, S. (1988). Bereavement groups: Techniques and themes. *International Journal of Group Psychology 38*(4), 419-446.

Young, D. (1987). Crisis in obstetrics—the management of labor. *International Journal of Childbirth Education 2*(3), 13-15

Index